# Brain Health
## ACROSS THE LIFE SPAN

PROCEEDINGS OF A WORKSHOP



Anna Nicholson, *Rapporteur*

Board on Population Health and Public Health Practice

Health and Medicine Division

*The National Academies of*
SCIENCES • ENGINEERING • MEDICINE

THE NATIONAL ACADEMIES PRESS
*Washington, DC*
**www.nap.edu**

**THE NATIONAL ACADEMIES PRESS 500 Fifth Street, NW Washington, DC 20001**

This activity was supported by the Department of Health and Human Services' Office of the Assistant Secretary for Health. Any opinions, findings, conclusions, or recommendations expressed in this publication do not necessarily reflect the views of any organization or agency that provided support for the project.

International Standard Book Number-13: 978-0-309-67261-0
International Standard Book Number-10: 0-309-67261-9
Digital Object Identifier: https://doi.org/10.17226/25703

Additional copies of this publication are available from the National Academies Press, 500 Fifth Street, NW, Keck 360, Washington, DC 20001; (800) 624-6242 or (202) 334-3313; http://www.nap.edu.



Printed in the United States of America

Suggested citation: National Academies of Sciences, Engineering, and Medicine. 2020. *Brain health across the life span: Proceedings of a workshop*. Washington, DC: The National Academies Press. https://doi.org/10.17226/25703.

*The National Academies of*
# SCIENCES · ENGINEERING · MEDICINE

The **National Academy of Sciences** was established in 1863 by an Act of Congress, signed by President Lincoln, as a private, nongovernmental institution to advise the nation on issues related to science and technology. Members are elected by their peers for outstanding contributions to research. Dr. Marcia McNutt is president.

The **National Academy of Engineering** was established in 1964 under the charter of the National Academy of Sciences to bring the practices of engineering to advising the nation. Members are elected by their peers for extraordinary contributions to engineering. Dr. John L. Anderson is president.

The **National Academy of Medicine** (formerly the Institute of Medicine) was established in 1970 under the charter of the National Academy of Sciences to advise the nation on medical and health issues. Members are elected by their peers for distinguished contributions to medicine and health. Dr. Victor J. Dzau is president.

The three Academies work together as the **National Academies of Sciences, Engineering, and Medicine** to provide independent, objective analysis and advice to the nation and conduct other activities to solve complex problems and inform public policy decisions. The National Academies also encourage education and research, recognize outstanding contributions to knowledge, and increase public understanding in matters of science, engineering, and medicine.

Learn more about the National Academies of Sciences, Engineering, and Medicine at **www.nationalacademies.org.**

## PLANNING COMMITTEE ON BRAIN HEALTH ACROSS THE LIFE SPAN[1]

**HUDA AKIL,** Gardner Quarton Distinguished University Professor of Neuroscience and Psychiatry and Codirector of the Molecular & Behavioral Neuroscience Institute, University of Michigan
**B. J. CASEY,** Professor of Psychology, Adjunct Professor of Psychology in Psychiatry and Neuroscience, Yale University
**DAMIEN A. FAIR,** Associate Professor of Behavioral Neuroscience and Associate Professor of Psychiatry, Oregon Health & Science University
**JENNIFER J. MANLY,** Professor of Neuropsychology in Neurology at the Gertrude H. Sergievsky Center and the Taub Institute for Research in Aging and Alzheimer's Disease, Columbia University
**BRUCE S. McEWEN,** Alfred E. Mirsky Professor, The Rockefeller University
**BRUCE L. MILLER,** A.W. and Mary Margaret Clausen Distinguished Professor in Neurology, University of California, San Francisco

*Health and Medicine Division Staff*

**KATHLEEN STRATTON,** Scholar
**ROSE MARIE MARTINEZ,** Senior Board Director
**ANDREW MERLUZZI,** Program Officer
**ANNA MARTIN,** Administrative Assistant
**PAMELA RAMEY-McCRAY,** Senior Program Assistant (*until October 2019*)

*Consultant*

**ANNA NICHOLSON,** Science Writer

[1] The National Academies of Sciences, Engineering, and Medicine's planning committees are solely responsible for organizing the workshop, identifying topics, and choosing speakers. The responsibility for the published Proceedings of a Workshop rests with the workshop rapporteur and the institution.

# In Memoriam

This Proceedings of a Workshop is dedicated to Dr. Bruce S. McEwen, who served as a planning committee member for this project. Dr. McEwen's research transformed our understanding of how the brain changes throughout life, especially with respect to hormones, stress, and resilience. He was an elected member of the National Academy of Sciences and the National Academy of Medicine and a cherished friend to the National Academies of Sciences, Engineering, and Medicine as a whole. He will be dearly missed.

# Reviewers

This Proceedings of a Workshop was reviewed in draft form by individuals chosen for their diverse perspectives and technical expertise. The purpose of this independent review is to provide candid and critical comments that will assist the National Academies of Sciences, Engineering, and Medicine in making each published proceedings as sound as possible and to ensure that it meets the institutional standards for quality, objectivity, evidence, and responsiveness to the charge. The review comments and draft manuscript remain confidential to protect the integrity of the process.

We thank the following individuals for their review of this proceedings:

**LISBETH NIELSEN,** National Institute on Aging, National Institutes of Health
**MARTA SNYDER TAGGERT,** BrightFocus Foundation
**WILLIAM A. VEGA,** Florida International University

Although the reviewers listed above provided many constructive comments and suggestions, they were not asked to endorse the content of the proceedings nor did they see the final draft before its release. The review of this proceedings was overseen by **MARTÍN J. SEPÚLVEDA,** Claraluzz, LLC. He was responsible for making certain that an independent examination of this proceedings was carried out in accordance with standards of the National Academies and that all review comments were carefully considered. Responsibility for the final content rests entirely with the rapporteur and the National Academies.

# Contents

# Boxes, Figures, and Table

## BOXES



## FIGURES

## TABLE

# Acronyms and Abbreviations

| | |
|---|---|
| ABCD | Adolescent Brain Cognitive Development Study |
| ACC | anterior cingulate cortex |
| ACE | adverse childhood experience |
| ACTH | adrenocorticotropic hormone |
| ADHD | attention-deficit hyperactivity disorder |
| BMI | body mass index |
| CNS | central nervous system |
| CTR | control |
| DSM-5 | *Diagnostic and Statistical Manual of Mental Disorders, 5th Edition* |
| ECHO | Environmental Influences on Child Health Outcomes |
| EEG | electroencephalography |
| ER | endoplasmic reticulum |
| fMRI | functional magnetic resonance imaging |
| HHS | Department of Health and Human Services |
| HPA | hypothalamic–pituitary–adrenal |
| IGF1 | insulin-like growth factor 1 |
| IL | interleukin |

| | |
|---|---|
| IL-6 | interleukin-6 |
| IQ | intelligence quotient |
| MIDUS | Midlife in the United States study |
| MRI | magnetic resonance imaging |
| NIA | National Institute on Aging |
| NIH | National Institutes of Health |
| OCD | obsessive–compulsive disorder |
| PET | positron emission tomography |
| PNC | Philadelphia Neurodevelopmental Cohort |
| PPARG | peroxisome proliferator-activated receptor gamma |
| RDoC | Research Domain Criteria |
| REGARDS | Reasons for Geographic and Racial Differences in Stroke |
| SAF | Safe American Family |
| sCCA | sparse canonical correlation analysis |
| SCN | suprachiasmatic nucleus |
| SES | socioeconomic status |
| SPECT | single-photon emission computed tomography |
| STAI | State–Trait Anxiety Inventory |
| TPH2 | tryptophan-hydroxylase 2 |
| WHICAP | Washington Heights–Inwood Columbia Aging Project |
| WSD | Western-style diet |

# 1

# Introduction

In his welcoming remarks, Admiral Brett Giroir, assistant secretary for health at the Department of Health and Human Services (HHS), underscored the importance of improving brain health across the life span, from birth through old age. Brain health affects Americans across all ages, genders, races, and ethnicities. Enriching the body of scientific knowledge around brain health and cognitive ability has the potential to improve quality of life and longevity for many millions of Americans and their families. The Centers for Disease Control and Prevention estimate that as many as 5 million Americans were living with Alzheimer's disease in 2014. That same year, more than 800,000 children were treated for concussion or traumatic brain injuries in U.S. emergency departments. Each year, more than 795,000 people in the United States have a stroke. Developing more effective treatment strategies for brain injuries and illnesses is essential, but brain health is not focused exclusively on disease, disorders, and vulnerability. It is equally important to better understand the ways our brains grow, learn, adapt, and heal. Addressing all of these domains to optimize brain health will require consideration about how to define brain health and resilience and about how to identify key elements to measure those concepts. Understanding the interactions between the brain, the body, and socioenvironmental forces is also fundamental to improving brain health.

To promote the improvement of brain health for all Americans, this conversation must extend beyond the realm of public health. It is critical to bring together expertise across sectors—including researchers, health care providers, mental health experts, the business community, educators, first responders, military, law enforcement personnel, and athletes—to explore how the brain develops and changes throughout the life span. HHS is currently tackling issues related to brain health through its work in many different offices, including several projects within the Office of the Assistant Secretary for Health (see Box 1-1). Giroir said that HHS will work with the National Academies of Sciences, Engineering, and

**BOX 1-1**
**Office of Disease Prevention and Health Promotion Initiatives Related to Brain Health**

The Office of Disease Prevention and Health Promotion within the Office of the Assistant Secretary for Health of the Department of Health and Human Services has several ongoing initiatives with components related to brain health.

***Healthy People 2030*** is the latest iteration of an initiative that has been under way for many decades, setting forth goals and objectives to improve the health of the country. It provides a road map for health promotion and disease prevention that includes multiple brain health objectives and goals over time. The previous version, ***Healthy People 2020***, looked at issues such as traumatic brain injury, suicide, depression, substance use disorder, severe mental illness, dementia, and cognitive decline as well as developmental screening for young people.

The ***Physical Activity Guidelines for Americans*** (second edition) was released in 2018 at the American Heart Association annual meeting. The 2018 Physical Activity Advisory Committee helped develop the science base for this policy. The guidelines offer evidence-based guidance about physical activity, health promotion, and prevention of chronic diseases. Habitual physical activity has many positive effects on brain health. The Physical Activity Guidelines Advisory Committee showed that habitual physical activity reduces symptoms of anxiety and depression, lowers the risks of developing depression and dementia, and helps to improve sleep quality. Individuals who habitually perform physical activities usually report having a better quality of life. Acute physical activity has also been shown to decrease anxiety in adults and to increase certain aspects of cognition in youths.

The ***Dietary Guidelines for Americans*** is released by the office every 5 years and is updated as nutrition science evolves. A 2020 Dietary Guidelines Advisory Committee is evaluating how components of diet are linked to brain health. For example, it is looking at how various dietary patterns consumed at different stages of life may influence neurocognitive development and health.

The office co-hosted a Healthy Aging Summit in 2018 and is convening a series of regional workshops around the country in anticipation of the next Healthy Aging Summit in 2021.

SOURCE: As presented by Richard Olson, director of the Division of Prevention Science at the Office of Disease Prevention and Health Promotion at the workshop Brain Health Across the Life Span on September 24, 2019.

Medicine to host a companion workshop focused on bringing these voices to the table and outlining ways that key sectors of society can apply the latest scientific evidence to educate the public about brain health. This work will help to ensure that America is positioned to lead the world in advancing the science, policies, and programs to improve brain health across the age spectrum, from premature infancy through old age.

## WORKSHOP OBJECTIVES

To explore issues related to brain health throughout the life span, from birth through old age, a public workshop titled Brain Health Across the Life Span was convened on September 24 and 25, 2019, by the Board on Population Health and Public Health Practice in the Health and Medicine Division of the National Academies. The workshop was sponsored by the Office of the Assistant Secretary for Health. The workshop was structured into seven sessions held over 2 days, featuring invited presentations and discussions that focused on the following questions:

- What are accepted definitions of brain health and resilience?
- What are the key elements to measure the status of brain health and its resilience across the life span?
- What additional research questions can be addressed to increase our understanding of brain plasticity throughout the life span?

In accordance with the policies of the National Academies, the workshop did not attempt to establish any conclusions or develop recommendations about needs and future directions, focusing instead on issues identified by the speakers and workshop participants. In addition, the organizing committee's role was limited to planning the workshop. This workshop proceedings was prepared by workshop rapporteur Anna Nicholson as a factual summary of what occurred at the workshop.

## ORGANIZATION OF THE PROCEEDINGS

This Proceedings of a Workshop is organized into seven chapters based on the order of topics presented at the workshop. The overall workshop was structured to begin with definitions and then broaden the scope to discuss brain health in various contexts. Throughout the workshop, participants generated definitions and ways to measure brain health and resilience, which are discussed throughout the Proceedings. Chapter 2 provides an overview of the fundamentals of brain health and resilience, specifically focused on how to define these terms. Recognizing that brain health and resilience cannot be defined in isolation, Chapter 3 looks at the role of brain–body interactions in brain health, while Chapter 4 explores the convergence of biology and behavior. Chapter 5 provides methodological insights for measuring brain health at many levels, and describes possible pathways toward precision neuroscience. Chapter 6 broadens the discussion further, examining brain health in the social context. Chapter 7 explores brain health across the life span, with a focus on ways forward in brain health measurement and research. The planning committee biographies can be found in Appendix A, the agenda for the workshop is in Appendix B, and the references are found in Appendix C.

# 2

# Fundamentals of Brain Health and Resilience

**Key Points Highlighted by Workshop Participants**

- A comprehensive approach takes into account individual, family, and social contexts as well as the elemental parts of the brain that are critical to its functioning, including neural circuits, neural cells, genes, and epigenetic modifications. A core concept is the process of bidirectional regulation: each of these levels modulates each of the other levels. (Huda Akil)
- Brain resilience is not just the absence of vulnerability, and brain resilience requires some exposure to stress. (Huda Akil)
- Efforts to characterize brain health should be framed by specifically defined outcomes and endpoints. For example, in addition to addressing cognitive decline and other issues related to mental health and aging, outcomes could also include such targets as improving quality of life. (Damien Fair)
- To enhance the precision of defining and measuring brain health, it is important to quantify and capture dimensions of life quality, well-being, purpose, social connection, and other related factors. (Lis Nielsen)

This chapter features a summary of the opening remarks by Huda Akil, codirector and research professor of the Molecular and Behavioral Neuroscience Institute and Quarton Professor of Neurosciences at the University of Michigan. Akil set the stage for the workshop by describing a multiscale approach for brain health, which was followed by a discussion about how to define the concepts of brain health and resilience.

## MULTISCALE APPROACH FOR BRAIN HEALTH

Akil explained that the multiscale approach to understanding brain health and functioning does not merely consider the brain in isolation. Rather, this approach takes into account individual, family, and social contexts as well as the elemental parts of the brain that are critical to its functioning, including neural circuits, neural cells, genes, and epigenetic modifications. A core concept is the process of bidirectional regulation: each of these levels modulates all the other levels. This approach was originally developed as a model for brain disease, but it is equally relevant to brain health in considering how these biological, social, and environmental interactions work forward and backward to ensure greater health across all these levels of analysis.

The brain is extremely complex, comprising trillions of connections facilitated by neurotransmitters operating through neural networks. The field of neuroscience has developed a host of specialized tools for studying the brain, but this knowledge about how the brain functions needs to be translated into actionable ways to maintain and improve brain health. Akil listed three essential requirements of brain function:

1. The brain needs to control the body—including the brain itself—hence the importance of brain–body interactions.
2. The brain needs to monitor the outside world, hence the importance of both the physical and social contexts and how they affect the brain.
3. Given the complexity of the world, the brain needs to learn from experience. Physical change via learning is a quintessential, distinctive feature of the function of the mammalian brain, not merely a side effect.

"Nowadays our brains are unhappy with us, because our brains have evolved to handle a life that's quite different from the one we're living," said Akil. Humans' general health has been affected by modern society in new ways, with the brain being either the primary site or a major target of these disruptions. How people use their brains has changed as the world becomes increasingly complex and demanding. The availability of more options and choices has been tempered with a reduced sense of predictability and control, which are major drivers of stress. Furthermore, humans are social animals, but social support systems have changed dramatically in the modern world. At the same time, the human life span has increased, and the expectations associated with each stage of life have expanded. Because people live longer, more complicated lives, their brains need to stay healthy longer.

Akil emphasized the importance of finding ways to compensate for these lifestyle changes by helping human brains adapt in positive ways. She posited that the huge global burden of brain disorders is a manifestation of this disconnection between the way people live today and the ways human brains have adapted. Increases in depression and other mood disorders, suicide, autism, dementia, Alzheimer's disease, and other neurodegenerative disorders, and the epidemics of opioid misuse and other substance use disorders, may all be signs that our brains are unhappy with us. This gives rise to the question of how to achieve greater health both for disease prevention and for human happiness more broadly. The goal of this multiscale approach to brain health is to make people healthier and more aware of how their brains function, thus providing them with a sense of power over the brain and a sense of hope that they will be able to cope with challenges.

## FUNDAMENTAL CONCEPTS OF BRAIN HEALTH AND RESILIENCE

The absence of standardized definitions for the terms "resilience" and "brain health" was a common refrain at the workshop. In order to provide context for the workshop's presentations and discussions, Akil outlined a set of fundamental concepts related to brain health and resilience. Each person's brain is unique; because of this brain diversity, there is no single or universal way to achieve brain health. People have multiple coping and learning styles, they live in a variety of contexts and social settings, and they use an array of tools and strategies. Therefore, a diversity of approaches will be needed to help people become more resilient. A consequent consideration is the challenge of measuring brain health in the context of this degree of diversity. Most brain disorders result from interactions between genes and the environment. Although this makes the disorders complicated to study, the environmental component provides opportunities for prevention. This can begin early in life by providing children with rich physical and social environments. Identifying opportunities for prevention will require identifying the essential features of an environment that promote brain health across different ages and stages.

The concept of resilience is often thought of as an intrinsic quality, similar to a rubber band that stretches and rebounds back into its original shape. However, in the context of brain health, resilience is not an inbuilt quality; being resilient does not mean never having been vulnerable in the first place. Rather, the brain has mechanisms to build resilience—called counter-regulatory mechanisms—that develop to combat distress. Akil described the relationship between vulnerability and resilience as "yin and yang" in the sense that the development of resilience requires some exposure to stress. This gives rise to questions about how to differentiate good stress—which can help to build resilience—from bad stress, which is ongoing chronic stress. It is important to minimize the lifelong allostatic load of stress so it does not begin to damage the brain.

The concept of neuroplasticity refers to the brain's ability to remodel itself. This is not just an ephemeral concept, but an active process of physical remodeling of brain structure and function. New cells are born, new connections are formed, and branches broaden. However, neuroplasticity is not an infinite resource. The concept of metaplasticity shows that there are limits on the extent to which the brain can be remodeled. For example, if remodeling in the brain occurs to cope with opioid addiction, then the ability to remodel the brain to cope with depression is limited. As with stress, neuroplasticity can be good or bad; therefore, it is important to support "good" neuroplasticity and use it wisely.

Brain remodeling is an ongoing process that must adapt to different demands throughout the life span, Akil noted. During critical periods—such as early development, adolescence, and menopause—molecular programming opens the system to more extensive remodeling. A major challenge is maintaining this remodeling capacity with advanced age. An associated question is how to foster and maintain this remodeling ability throughout the life span by taking advantage of windows of opportunity and providing lifelong support.

Akil invited workshop participants to reflect on the relationship between brain health and resilience, as well as their own definitions of those two concepts. Lis Nielsen, chief of the Individual Behavioral Processes Branch of the Division of Behavioral and Social Research at the National Institute on Aging (NIA), commented on NIA's ongoing efforts to examine the potential for plasticity in midlife or later life to reverse or compensate for risks associated with early-life adversity. The shaping of brain health begins very early in the life span—perhaps even earlier when accounting for intergenerational influences—and this underscores the need to consider individual differences in brain health trajectories. These include biological embedding of the social environment as well as the potential for particular kinds of interventions to promote positive plasticity, depending on an individual's life history and exposures throughout the life span. In the context of resilience, individuals may carry multiple life histories and imprinting of extreme adverse exposures. However, positive imprinting may be possible as well. Akil added that the environment can affect the way a person's genome functions, with some evidence suggesting that this effect is even transmitted between generations and is thus not easily reversible. This underscores the need to find ways to counterbalance the epigenetic intergenerational effect.

Damien Fair, associate professor of behavioral neuroscience, associate professor of psychiatry, and associate scientist at the Advanced Imaging Research Center at the Oregon Health & Science University, remarked that efforts to characterize brain health should be framed by specifically defined outcomes and endpoints that are being targeted. For example, in addition to addressing cognitive decline and other issues related to mental health and aging, outcomes could also include such targets as improving quality of life. Akil suggested that the absence of disease or disorders is a potential way to define brain health.

Molly Wagster, NIA, said that at the third Cognitive Aging Summit in 2017, participants highlighted the lack of uniformity across the research community in their definitions of fundamental concepts and constructs such as brain reserve, cognitive reserve, resilience, resistance, and compensation. One of the recommendations generated by the summit was to operationalize these concepts—that is, clearly define what is meant by each of those concepts, how to measure them, and in what contexts they do and do not apply. As a result, a group of researchers from across disciplines related to brain health is currently working to develop consistent definitions of relevant terms. To enhance the precision of this work, Nielsen suggested drawing from the rich body of research around quantifying and capturing the dimensions of life quality, well-being, purpose, social connection, and other related factors. It is also important to contextualize subjective well-being across subpopulations who may prioritize different aspects of well-being or have different opportunities for attaining well-being, she said. For example, some people have greater opportunities to live a purposeful, goal-striving life and tend to rate that dimension as the most important for their well-being. People who lack those kinds of opportunities may rate merely enjoying the pleasures of daily social interactions as being the most important dimension.

Akil noted that there is a dearth of research on the biology of joy and happiness in the brain beyond neuroscientific work on immediate reward. However, the field of positive psychology looks at different ways people can achieve a sense of fulfillment. This ranges from living a good life internally, to feeling engaged, and to having a purpose. She pointed to a large research gap in understanding how the brain of a person who is living a purposeful life compares with a person who is not, for example, or the differences between the brain of a person who reports feeling active joy—not just contentment—on a regular basis, and that of a person who does not. She reiterated that resilience should not be defined simply as absence of vulnerability, but instead be defined as an "affective algebra." The positives and negatives need to be balanced such that the algebra comes out on the positive side.

Akil urged the participants to consider ways to understand and quantify resilience on a biological level within and across individuals. One strategy might be to study the brain, behavior, biology, and contexts of people who report feeling good about their life despite major adversities, like being paralyzed or having a sick child. Fair added that the crux of the research agenda should be to work toward precise, reliable measurements to integrate the research being done by people working across the scientific spectrum, such as by integrating work on joy and happiness with work on brain biology.

# 3

# Brain–Body Interactions

**Key Points Highlighted by Workshop Participants**

- Coordinating and standardizing measurements for better reliability as well as validity and cross-comparisons will be important for measuring brain health. (Huda Akil)
- Stress is a multinomial construct; studies tend to focus only on stress that leads to negative outcomes, while the notion of positive stress is often overlooked in research. This is a research gap that must be addressed. (Natalie Rasgon)
- Brain diseases—as with many "body" diseases—are not discrete events in time. They may develop as a continuum and accumulation. Research should focus less on drawing distinct lines and more on describing the continuum of brain health. (Natalie Rasgon)
- Decisions about how to define the presence of disease can be avoided by moving toward a preventive, long-term, life-course perspective. This would focus on resilience, restorative processes, and the potential to achieve positive health by mitigating risk factors or early exposures. (Lis Nielsen)

This chapter summarizes the presentations and panel discussion from the workshop session on brain–body interactions. The session focused on how the brain interacts with the body and the implications these interactions have for measuring and maximizing brain health and resilience. Evidence from research on brain–body interactions demonstrates the importance of this connection and suggests possible avenues for future research on brain health. Colleen McClung, professor of psychiatry and clinical and translational science at the University of Pittsburgh, described the effect of circadian rhythms on health across the life span. The relationship between early environmental risk factors and mental health disorders was explored by Elinor Sullivan, associate professor at the University of Oregon. Natalie Rasgon, professor of psychiatry and behavioral sciences at the Stanford University Medical Center, explained how insulin resistance serves as a link in brain–body interaction.

## EFFECT OF CIRCADIAN RHYTHMS ON HEALTH ACROSS THE LIFE SPAN

McClung gave a presentation on the effect of circadian rhythms on brain and body health across the life span. Circadian rhythms change over the life span and contribute to different diseases at different stages of life, starting from early fetal development all the way through to old

### BOX 3-1
### Role of the Suprachiasmatic Nucleus in Coordinating Circadian Rhythms

Circadian rhythms are coordinated centrally in the brain by the suprachiasmatic nucleus (SCN), which receives light input directly from retinal ganglion cells in the eye. When the eye senses light—particularly the blue light spectrum—special photoreceptors carry that input into the brain. McClung likened the SCN to a "conductor of the orchestra" of the peripheral rhythms throughout the brain and body. Each cell in the body has circadian genes, but the SCN coordinates those rhythms in a variety of ways. For instance, the SCN controls the release of hormones such as melatonin—which is released at night and helps to promote sleep—and cortisol, a hormone released in the morning that helps to promote wakefulness. In addition to entrainment by light, body clocks can be entrained by other environmental factors. The SCN also coordinates body temperature rhythms that synchronize the metabolic clocks throughout the other organs in the body, which can be set apart from the circadian clock in the brain by other factors, such as meal timing, for example.

SOURCE: As presented by Colleen McClung at the workshop Brain Health Across the Life Span on September 24, 2019.

age. Box 3-1 details how circadian rhythms are coordinated centrally in the brain by the suprachiasmatic nucleus (SCN). She explained that across a 24-hour day, circadian rhythms are prominent in every process in the body, including coordination, alertness, reaction time, cardiovascular activity, body temperature, and sleep. Disease symptoms and processes also appear to have circadian rhythms that revolve around the 24-hour cycle. For example, heart attacks are more common in the morning, while symptoms of restless leg syndrome typically occur in the evening; gout attacks occur mostly in the middle of the night, whereas stomach ulcers tend to occur in the middle of the day.

### Evolution of Circadian Rhythms Over the Life Span

Circadian rhythms evolve and change across a person's life span, noted McClung. These rhythms are shaped initially during the very early stages of development. At the beginning of the life span, a mother's circadian rhythms influence the development of fetal circadian rhythms, including tissue homeostasis and neurodevelopment as well as the development and consolidation of feeding, metabolic, and sleep–wake rhythms. Evidence is emerging that disruptions to a mother's circadian rhythms during pregnancy caused by shift work, for example, can have a long-term effect on the offspring (Logan and McClung, 2019).

Infants typically do not have a regular sleep–wake pattern—they usually sleep every 2 or 3 hours and eat whenever they are hungry. Patterns begin to coalesce in early childhood, and then a person's circadian rhythms undergo substantial changes during adolescence and into adulthood. After entering puberty, adolescents tend to undergo a shift in their circadian rhythms from an early to a late chronotype[1] (Roenneberg et al., 2004). For adolescents who must wake very early for school, this shift can create a sense of circadian misalignment and sleep loss that is similar to jet lag and puts stress on the adolescent brain. As people age, their rhythm gradually shifts back toward an earlier chronotype.

Melatonin secretion also changes over the life span (Grivas and Savvidou, 2007). Newborns have very little melatonin secretion, but it increases sharply and peaks during the early childhood and preteen years. Melatonin secretion begins to decline around puberty and continues to decrease through middle age to minimal secretion during old age. For older people, this loss of melatonin contributes to a loss of synchrony

[1] "Chronotype" refers to how an individual's circadian clock synchronizes or entrains to the 24-hour day (Roenneberg et al., 2004).

of circadian rhythms, and, because melatonin is an effective antioxidant, it may also contribute to neural degeneration later in life.

A person's specific individual genotype also contributes to circadian rhythms. For example, most people shift back from the late-night phenotype after adolescence, others remain "late night" people for the rest of their lives. Many people have regular, normal sleep phases (roughly in the window of 10 p.m. to 8 a.m.), but others have delayed sleep phase (sleeping from 4 a.m. to 12 p.m.) or advanced sleep phase (5 p.m. to 3 a.m.). Still others have irregular sleep–wake patterns or a non-24-hour sleep–wake rhythm. The latter is experienced by people who cannot entrain to the environment—owing to blindness, dementia, cognitive impairment, or mental disorders, for example—such that their rhythms shift slightly each day.

In addition to genetic changes in circadian rhythms or differences in circadian rhythms, the modern lifestyle has markedly influenced our circadian clocks. Artificial lighting at night disrupts normal circadian rhythms, as do shift work, travel across time zones, eating late at night, and consuming caffeine, alcohol, and other drugs. Dim lighting in the morning is incompatible with the way human brains evolved based on sun exposure during the morning and sleeping in darkness at night. These lifestyle factors can have serious consequences for brain health and body health.

## Circadian Desynchrony Contributes to Different Diseases at Different Stages of Life

Whether it is caused by genetic or environmental factors or both, circadian desynchrony contributes to a variety of conditions, including brain diseases that have circadian rhythms at their core, such as bipolar disorder, major depression, drug addiction, and schizophrenia (Kasper et al., 2018). Because every organ has a circadian rhythm, circadian disruption also affects metabolism, obesity, diabetes, cancer, and cardiac health.

### *Addiction*

Childhood and adolescent sleep characteristics can predict later substance abuse. Studies have associated a variety of substance abuse outcomes in teenagers and young adults with different types of sleep and circadian disturbances, such as sleep quality, sleepiness, evening preference, and weekend delays in sleeping patterns (see Figure 3-1). Teenagers that experience a strong shift toward the evening chronotype during adolescence tend to have lower prefrontal cortical activation in response to reward, which correlates significantly with alcohol consumption (Hasler

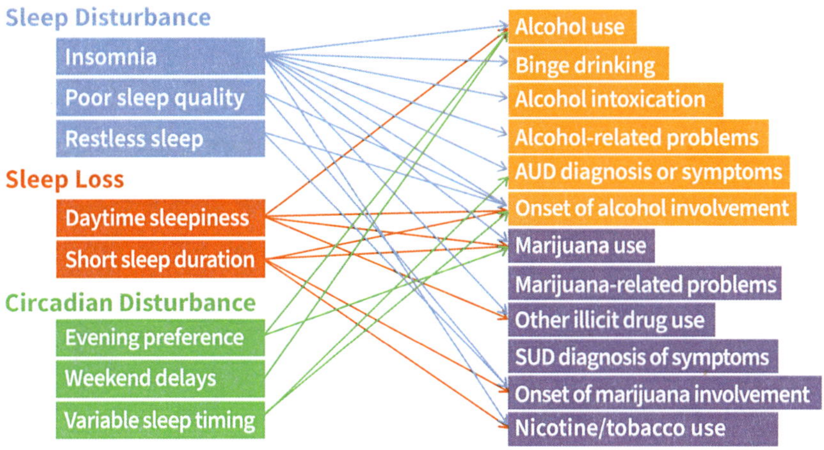


**FIGURE 3-1** Childhood and adolescent sleep characteristics predict later substance abuse.
NOTE: AUD = alcohol use disorder; SUD = substance use disorder.
SOURCES: As presented by Colleen McClung at the workshop Brain Health Across the Life Span on September 24, 2019 (courtesy of Dr. Brant Hasler).

et al., 2013). This loss of top-down control tends to make them greater risk takers and increases the likelihood of impulsive activities, such as drug and alcohol consumption (Hasler et al., 2013). The ventral striatal response—the reward center of the brain—increases among people who are evening types, which is associated with greater alcohol dependence in young adults and teenagers. It has been posited that evening-type teenagers who are required to wake up very early in the morning are losing sleep because they cannot get to sleep at night, so they sleep very late on the weekends. This constant state of circadian misalignment and sleep deprivation contributes to increased risk for substance abuse.

### *Psychiatric Disorders*

People with psychiatric disorders are profoundly influenced by changes in the circadian clock. Major disruption to the sleep and activity cycle is a common characteristic of disorders such as depression, bipolar disorder, schizophrenia, autism, and attention-deficit hyperactivity disorder (ADHD). In fact, bipolar disorder is becoming characterized as a circadian rhythm disorder, as schedule changes caused by international travel or night shift work can precipitate manic episodes, depressive episodes, or psychotic episodes. Depression is diurnal (i.e., worse in the morning), it is often seasonal, and it tends to occur more frequently in areas of the world where there is little daylight for long periods of time. People with a preference toward "eveningness" are more susceptible to depression and make up the majority of people with bipolar disorder. Polymorphisms in several circadian genes associate with psychiatric disorders in humans and mice, and evidence has shown that circadian gene mutations have many phenotypes that resemble depression and bipolar disorder. Furthermore, evidence from genetic studies and animal studies suggests that circadian genes are directly involved in modulating mood and reward.

### *Animal Studies*

Experimental shifting of animals' light–dark cycles can lead to increased tumors. A mouse model of cancer has demonstrated that putting the animals on a shift-work cycle increases tumor growth, the number of tumors, and tumor aggressiveness (Logan et al., 2012). Mouse studies demonstrate that mutation in the core circadian genes leads to weight gain on a regular diet and to obesity on a high-fat diet, attributable to loss of circadian rhythm in the genes and peptides involved in metabolic control (Turek et al., 2005). Furthermore, a high-fat diet itself can disrupt behavioral and molecular circadian rhythms in mice, even in the absence of genetic mutation. A poor diet leads to irregular circadian rhythmicity in mice, especially in the fat and in the liver, which also contributes to weight gain. This is a vicious cycle of disrupting circadian rhythms with unhealthy food intake, with those circadian rhythms also influencing metabolic rates (Kohsaka et al., 2007). Recent research has focused on using timed restricted feeding to control this effect. Because mice are nocturnal, restricting their feeding to nighttime causes increased amplitude of rhythms and fewer problems with the metabolic system compared with mice who eat at various times of the day (Hatori et al., 2012).

### *Neurodegeneration*

In older people with neurodegeneration, circadian rhythm disruption may increase the progression of neuronal loss, may lead to earlier loss of cognitive function, and may be related to accumulation of amyloid-beta and tau (Musiek, 2017). Figure 3-2 illustrates how this represents yet another vicious cycle: Alzheimer's disease and other neurodegenerative diseases affect the circadian clock, while the circadian clock influences inflammation, oxidation, and endoplasmic reticulum (ER) stress, all of which worsen the brain disease and its progression (Chauhan et al., 2017).

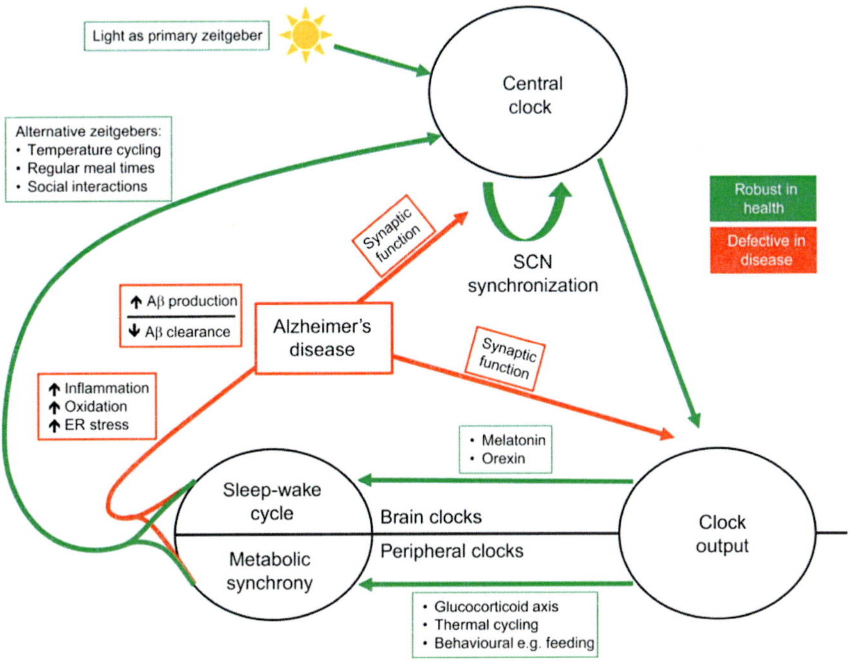


**FIGURE 3-2** Vicious cycle of circadian rhythm disruption and neurodegeneration.
NOTES: "Zeitgeber" refers to a rhythmically occurring phenomenon that acts as a break in the regulation of circadian rhythm. Aβ = amyloid-beta; ER = endoplasmic reticulum; SCN = suprachiasmatic nucleus.
SOURCES: As presented by Colleen McClung at the workshop Brain Health Across the Life Span on September 24, 2019; Chauhan et al., 2017.

### Monitoring Circadian Rhythms as a Diagnostic Tool

Circadian rhythms can easily be monitored as a diagnostic tool and might be helpful in determining who is at risk for certain diseases or for monitoring the progression of diseases such as bipolar disorder, said McClung. A person's circadian rhythms can be understood by using a range of measures: activity and sleep patterns, cycling hormones (melatonin and cortisol), body temperature rhythms, peripheral circadian gene expression (blood, saliva, and buccal cells), and cycling metabolites (urine). Actigraphy is an easy-to-use technique for assessing a person's sleep–wake patterns using a noninvasive wearable sensor, similar in size to a wristwatch, that automatically determines the person's sleep–wakefulness state. This simple, low-cost solution can be used to gather valuable information and allow for long-term monitoring. For example, physicians can be trained to monitor the activity patterns of a person with bipolar disorder or depression in order to recognize the onset of manic or depressive episodes and prompt a therapeutic intervention.

### Strategies for Stabilizing Circadian Rhythms

McClung explained that circadian rhythms can be stabilized to both help and prevent disease in a number of ways, through either environmental or pharmacological stabilization. Natural strategies that people can use to stabilize their own rhythms include the following:

- Spending at least 20 to 30 minutes in natural morning sunlight
- Using a light therapy bulb or lamp if indoors all day
- Avoiding brightly lit screens for at least 1 hour before bed
- Going to bed at the same time every night and waking at same time each day
- Sleeping in complete darkness
- Restricting meals primarily to daytime (e.g., no late-night snacking)

The technology for measuring rhythms and for helping people with rhythm analysis and stabilization is improving. Mobile applications have been developed to track a person's circadian rhythms, detect light, and recommend how much light the person needs (Wehr, 2018). Another application developed at the University of Michigan helps to entrain people before they travel overseas, by telling them when to take melatonin and when to get light. A technique called social rhythm therapy has been developed primarily for people with bipolar disorder by Ellen Frank and colleagues at the University of Pittsburgh, through which clinicians can intervene using a very strict sleep–wake schedule. In people with bipolar disorder who have disruptive locomotor rhythms, social rhythm therapy can improve their sleep–wake cycles and stabilize their moods. Daily bright light therapy between 12 p.m. and 2:30 p.m. has been shown to help people with bipolar depression (Sit et al., 2018).

Pharmacotherapies such as lithium and valproic acid—two first-line treatments for bipolar disorder—can enhance circadian rhythm amplitude (Johansson et al., 2011; Li et al., 2012). Pharmaceutical companies are working to develop medications that will target the circadian clock specifically to create the amplification of circadian rhythms but without the other numerous side effects that lithium and valproic acid can cause. This may represent the next wave of interventions to enhance circadian rhythms and prevent or treat diseases.

## Leveraging Circadian Rhythms to Optimize Treatment

Current treatments for a variety of diseases can take advantage of rhythms to optimize the time of day for greatest effect, said McClung. For example, a cluster-randomized trial found that influenza vaccination in the morning enhances antibody response more than afternoon vaccination because the immune system is primed in the morning (Long et al., 2016). Similarly, taking statins to treat heart disease at a particular time of day achieves a better effect, while birth control pills need to be taken at the same time of day every day to be highly effective. This technique is now being used in in chemotherapy because tumors tend to have a different circadian rhythm than the surrounding cells (Levi et al., 2007). By using a chemotherapy agent that attacks cells at a specific stage of the cell cycle, it is possible to maximize the effect on tumor cells while minimizing the effect on the surrounding cells if the treatment is delivered at the appropriate time of day.

## Discussion

Huda Akil, codirector and research professor of the Molecular and Behavioral Neuroscience Institute and Quarton Professor of Neurosciences at the University of Michigan, asked McClung to elaborate on how early-life patterns can predict behavior much later in life. She replied that the studies are in the early stages, but mouse models indicate that disrupting the rhythms of pregnant mice with a protocol similar to shift work has an effect on the risk-taking and reward-related behavior later in life in the offspring mice. Although the underlying mechanism is not yet understood, females seem to be more susceptible than males, which indicates that it may be related to hormones in some way.

Rasgon commented that light therapy is useful when appropriately used in mood disorders and in patients with neurodegenerative disease, especially in dementia patients who exhibit sundowning syndrome[2] or circadian-induced delirium. She asked if light therapy or some kind of sensory induction could promote a certain stabilization of the consciousness. McClung replied that there have not yet been many clinical studies to determine if changing circadian rhythms in these patients will improve their outcomes. However, research carried out in nursing home and hospital environments with variable light environments (e.g., dim levels of light that persist into the night) have found that exposure to very bright lights during the day and darkness during the night can improve

[2] Sundowning refers to restlessness, aggression, anxiety, or other behavioral issues that can happen in the evening in patients with some forms of dementia, including Alzheimer's disease.

cognition and perhaps even reduce sundowning, which is a common problem in dementia patients that can be a challenge to caregivers as well. Akil noted that there are certain wavelengths in sunrise and sunset that are important for setting the circadian rhythms, but those wavelengths are not completely captured by current lighting therapies.

A participant asked for clarification about how the decrease in melatonin may contribute to neurodegenerative diseases. McClung replied that data suggest that melatonin is protective in neurodegenerative disorders such as Huntington's disease and amyotrophic lateral sclerosis. Melatonin is a signaling hormone in the mitochondria and acts as a potent antioxidant. Although the decline of melatonin over the life span is a natural biological process, the extent of the decrease varies by individual. Melatonin therapy also has the potential to help prevent or at least delay certain neurodegenerative diseases, she added.

## EARLY ENVIRONMENTAL RISK FACTORS FOR MENTAL HEALTH DISORDERS

Elinor Sullivan explored how the early environment influences both brain health and the risk of mental health disorders later in life. Multiple prenatal factors are associated with risk for mental health disorders, she explained. These include known factors, such as toxicant exposure and teratogens, but maternal obesity, maternal depression, poor maternal nutrition, and increased maternal stress have also been linked to increased risk of mental health disorders for the offspring. Her presentation focused largely on the factors of maternal obesity and poor maternal nutrition. Maternal obesity has long been shown to be associated with increased risk for childhood and adult obesity as well as metabolic disease. More recent evidence indicates that maternal obesity is also associated with risk for children developing anxiety, autism spectrum disorder, ADHD, emotional difficulties, cognitive problems, and eating disorders.

### Animal Model Studies of Early Environmental Exposures

Sullivan described how a nonhuman primate model has been used to help disentangle the comorbidity of these early environmental exposures by looking at how maternal obesity and Western-style diet (WSD) affect mental health–related behavior. The study design included two adult Japanese macaque breeding groups: one group remained on the control (CTR) diet and the other was placed on a high-fat WSD constructed to mimic the average American diet, which is high in saturated fat, high in caloric density, and high in sugar. Adult females were metabolically characterized in their nonpregnant and (third-trimester) pregnant states to assess adiposity, glucose metabolism, and insulin response. To mimic what happens in humans, the adult female macaques were placed on a WSD about 2 years prior to pregnancy and kept on the diet during gestation and lactation.

As with humans, the animals who consumed the average American diet tended to be heavier, to have increases in adiposity in response to the diet, and to have increases in their insulin area under the curve, suggesting that they were less sensitive to insulin and had a slight impairment in glucose regulation. In the control group, most of the animals had a lean body fat of 10–15 percent, although some animals drifted up to body fat of 30–35 percent. When animals were placed on a WSD, the histogram shifted. Some animals remained at a healthy 10–15 percent body fat, but many more fell within the 30–35 percent range and others moved into the 40–45 percent fat for their adiposity. This allowed the investigators to look at the offspring based on the mother's diet and her metabolic state as separate variables.

The offspring were weaned and subdivided into four groups:

1. CTR/CTR offspring who stayed on the mother's CTR diet
2. WSD/WSD offspring who stayed on the mother's WSD
3. CTR/WSD offspring whose mothers ate the CTR diet, but the offspring were switched to the WSD
4. WSD/CTR offspring whose mothers ate the WSD, but the offspring were switched to the CTR diet

The initial findings from this model pertain to anxiety-related behaviors in 4-month-old infants as manifested in their latency[3] to explore three different novel objects of varying levels of potential threat (Sullivan et al., 2010). Males and females whose mothers ate the CTR diet would touch novel objects rapidly, as did male offspring of mothers on the WSD. However, female offspring of mothers who ate the WSD had increased latency to interact with all three novel objects. Thus, maternal WSD consumption leads to increased latency to explore novel objects in female offspring, suggesting that the offspring have increased anxiety compared to the other groups.

To characterize this behavior in more detail, the investigators looked at the effect of maternal WSD exposure on offspring anxiety at 11 months (Thompson et al., 2017). A novel object test using a human intruder was used to assess the offspring's temperament relating to anxiety and depression. Among the offspring of mothers who consumed the WSD, increases

[3] "Latency" refers to the time between a stimulus and a response, in this case the time between presentation of the objects and exploration of the objects.

were seen in both the number of occurrences and the percent of test time that the animals engaged in anxiety behavior. Placing those offspring on the CTR diet at weaning did not ameliorate the changes—in fact, it slightly intensified the differences in anxiety behavior in these animals. An increase in stress-related vocalization was also seen in animals exposed to the WSD prenatally and an increase in active forms of anxiety, such as trying to escape from the cage, both in the number of occurrences and in the percent of test time. Male offspring who consumed a WSD after weaning showed increases in stereotypy. Therefore, some effects are different primarily by the mother's diet, while other behavioral effects seem to be driven by the offspring's current diet.

### *Possible Mechanisms for Behavioral Differences*

Sullivan said her group is exploring a set of mechanisms that may underlie the behavioral differences observed in the animal studies, including the following:

- Increased inflammation
- Maternal diet versus the maternal metabolic state
- Changes in the development of neurotransmitter systems critical in behavioral regulation
- Alterations in stress sensitivity as characterized by the hypothalamic–pituitary–adrenal axis
- Alterations in the early postnatal environment, such as maternal–infant behavior and attachment

A primary mechanism is increased inflammation. Chronic elevations in adiposity are associated with an increase in peripheral markers of inflammation. In their nonhuman primate model, the investigators were able to show that maternal WSD consumption resulted in increased developmental exposure to inflammatory cytokines. Increased microglial inflammation in the fetal hypothalamus suggests that the mother's inflammation affects the fetal environment and increases the offspring's exposure to inflammation. This is transmitted to the fetal brain, increasing neural inflammation, or at least microglial activation. The investigators believe that this inflammatory process in the brain affects the development of critical neurotransmitter systems.

Evidence suggests that maternal obesity and WSD consumption also influence the development of neural pathways that regulate behavior because of alterations in the serotonergic and dopamine systems. In the serotonergic system, for example, Sullivan and colleagues found that offspring exposed to a WSD during the prenatal and early postnatal periods showed a reduction in tryptophan-hydroxylase 2 (TPH2)[4] expression, suggesting that they were producing less serotonin (Sullivan et al., 2010). This hypothesis was supported by further research that revealed that the offspring from mothers who consumed a WSD had reduced amounts of serotonin in their cerebral spinal fluid (Thompson et al., 2017). By then characterizing the serotonin projection systems, the study found alterations in the frontopolar cortex (a region associated with complex, higher-order behavior). Similar studies are being conducted to explore the relationships between obesity, diet, serotonin, and serotonergic projections to the amygdala.

### Effect of Maternal Diet on Offspring Behavior

Sullivan provided an overview of her 2010 study's conclusions about the effect of a maternal WSD on offspring behavior. In nonhuman primates, maternal WSD and obesity impair offspring brain development and behavior, with offspring from WSD mothers at increased risk for developing behavioral disorders. Increased anxiety is seen in both male and female offspring, with earlier onset in females. Males in particular exhibited increased repetitive behaviors, with those increases driven by the mother's diet but also, more profoundly, by the offspring's current diet consumption. Male offspring also displayed increased aggression toward novel peers. When examining the offspring's social behaviors across settings, investigators saw signs of social withdrawal and impairments in social behavior among both male and female animals whose mothers consumed a WSD.

Sullivan outlined the potential programming mechanisms underpinning these behavioral alterations in WSD offspring. The WSD offspring have increased stress sensitivity, as evidenced by elevated cortisol across developmental time points that is almost double the levels found in the control offspring. WSD offspring have increased exposures to inflammation during development, as well as altered development of the serotonin system and changes in dopamine innervation of the prefrontal cortex. Anatomical and functional magnetic resonance imaging scanning studies have also revealed alterations in cortical–subcortical connectivity among this group. Changes in maternal behavior also contribute, with the WSD mothers nursing their infants more and grooming them less during the early stages of development; they also tend to retrieve their infants less frequently from dangerous situations.

To explore the effects of maternal diet versus metabolic state, researchers looked at specific behaviors and found that most behaviors were programmed by the mother's diet and nutrition (see Figure 3-3). However,

---

[4] TPH2 is the rate-limiting enzyme for serotonin synthesis expression in the dorsal assay.

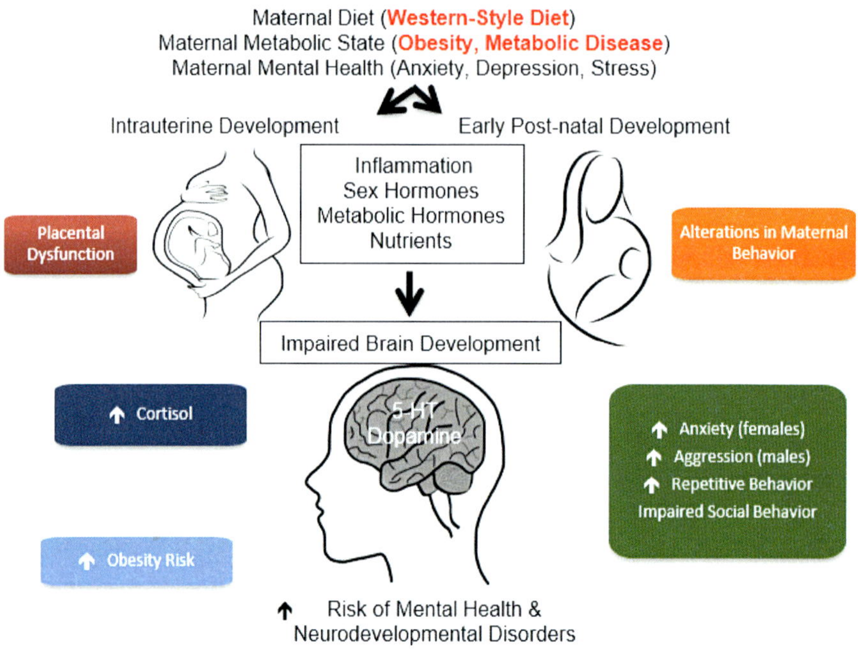


**FIGURE 3-3** Effect of maternal factors on offspring brain development and behavior.
SOURCES: As presented by Elinor Sullivan at the workshop Brain Health Across the Life Span on September 24, 2019; adapted from Rivera et al., 2015.

certain behaviors appear to be more strongly influenced by the maternal metabolic state. The investigators posit that both in nonhuman primates and in humans, the mother's diet, metabolic state, and mental health directly influence intrauterine development. The nonhuman primate model provides evidence for placental dysfunction and inflammation in the placenta, as indicated by less blood flow through the placenta of WSD mothers. Alterations in maternal behavior and direct effects on the early postnatal development are believed to occur through pathways such as inflammation and alterations in sex hormones, metabolic hormones, and nutrients. These factors come together to influence the way the brain is developing, Sullivan said. Thus far, investigators have found differences in the serotonin system and dopamine system, as well as changes in the melanocortin system that directly controls energy balance regulation. The primary behavioral outputs of anxiety, aggression, repetitive behaviors, and impaired social behavior are thought to be behavioral indicators of increased risk for mental health and neurodevelopmental disorders in humans, she added.

## Effect of Maternal Diet and Obesity on Offspring Risk for Neurodevelopmental Disorders

Sullivan explained that the investigators' next steps were to translate the findings from nonhuman primates into humans. Over the past decade, they have been characterizing mothers' diets and obesity and looking at their offspring's risk for neurodevelopmental disorders. Investigators began with a small pilot study looking at 68 mother–infant pairs and recently obtained National Institutes of Health (NIH) funding to recruit 300 participants; Sullivan presented preliminary data from the pilot study. The major study goals were to characterize the changes in the in utero environment associated with maternal obesity, poor nutrition, maternal stress, and maternal depression to determine which factors are the strongest predictors of alterations in infants' and toddlers' behaviors associated with ADHD and other neurodevelopmental disorders. Investigators are currently characterizing the infants and toddlers up to 3 years of age, and if their hypotheses are confirmed, they hope to develop new ideas for prevention and intervention to reduce neurodevelopmental disorders.

One of their first findings was that negative emotions are elevated in infants from families with ADHD. By looking at infants' affect at 6 months of age, investigators found that infants with a familial risk of ADHD (i.e., either one of their parents or a sibling was diagnosed with ADHD) showed early differences in how they interact in laboratory behavioral assessment tasks (Sullivan et al., 2015). Infants with a familial history of ADHD showed increased negative vocalizations during arm restraints and decreased attention-seeking regulatory behaviors during still-face paradigms. The same children are now 7 and 8 years of age, and the early 6-months-old measure strongly predicts the risk for ADHD, suggesting that this is an early biomarker for risk for ADHD.

The next focus of the study found that obesity was associated with increased inflammation during pregnancy in humans. As observed in the nonhuman primate study and reported in other literature, study participants who were obese had elevations in a series of cytokines, including interleukin-6 (IL-6), tumor necrosis-factor alpha, and monocyte-chemoattractant protein-1 (Gustafsson et al., 2019). Furthermore, maternal prepregnancy body mass index (BMI) and inflammatory profile were associated with higher negative emotionality among infants at 6 months of age. In addition to being related to familial risk of ADHD, offspring from obese mothers have also shown increased negative affect during the still-face paradigm, in which an adult expresses a neutral and unresponsive face toward an infant (Gustafsson et al., 2019). By probing this relationship further, investigators found that the relationship between maternal prepregnancy BMI and the 6-month-old infant's negative affect goes through inflammation—specifically, trimester IL-6 (Gustafsson et al., 2019). They believe that this inflammatory pathway, which was also observed in the nonhuman primates, is an important driver and represents another potential biomarker for increased risk for neurodevelopmental disorders.

When investigators added maternal nutrition into this relationship, they found that maternal prepregnancy BMI and fatty acid levels influence the child's negative affect. By looking at negative behaviors during the still-face paradigm and their relationship with prepregnancy BMI, negative behaviors increase as the mother's BMI increases (Gustafsson et al., 2019). If the mother's omega-3 fatty acid levels were one standard deviation below the mean of omega-3 fatty acids, this relationship was further exacerbated, with those offspring showing higher levels of negative behaviors. However, this relationship no longer held among mothers who were just one standard deviation above the mean of omega-3 fatty acids. Offspring whose mothers had an elevated prepregnancy body mass but were consuming higher levels of omega-3 fatty acid were actually protected from this effect. Sullivan emphasized that this is an optimistic finding, suggesting that some healthy foods can ameliorate some of the behavioral changes programmed by maternal obesity.

The investigators posit that inflammation is the common pathway to ADHD and other neurodevelopmental disorders. Omega-3 fatty acid was negatively associated with inflammation, maternal distress and depression were positively associated with inflammation, and maternal BMI was strongly associated with increased maternal inflammation. These factors were able to predict child ADHD symptoms at 4 to 6 years of age through the pathway of maternal inflammation.

## Future Research Directions

In addition to expanding the pilot study to validate findings in a larger cohort, the group's other ongoing studies will further examine inflammation as a mechanism in the breakdown of self-regulation and psychopathology. They will also explore the mechanisms for maternal nutrition-induced behavioral programming by looking at epigenetics, the microbiome, neuroimaging measures, and cell isolation and stimulation studies from the umbilical cord. The group's long-term goals are to develop clinical biomarkers of risks for neurodevelopmental disorders in order to develop early interventions. These may include dietary interventions (e.g., reduction in fat content and alterations in fat composition), exercise interventions, antioxidant treatments (e.g., resveratrol), and supplementation with critical amino acids (e.g., tryptophan). Thus far, the most promising finding is that omega-3 fatty acid consumption or supplementation could be an effective intervention. Ultimately, Sullivan's group aims to design effective prevention strategies as well.

### Discussion

Akil asked if features other than omega-3 fatty acid shortages or deficits contribute to the inflammatory process. Sullivan replied that all unrefined carbohydrates—but specifically sugar—and saturated fats are the two major drivers of this inflammation. Rather than total fat intake, it is likely the type of fat that is the concern. Omega-3 fatty acids are known to be protective, whereas elevated omega-6 fatty acids are helping to drive inflammation to some degree. With respect to unrefined carbohydrates, detailed nutrition measures in humans are already available that could be used to inform direct testing of those relationships in nonhuman primate models. When asked about any interaction between familial ADHD vulnerability and maternal obesity, Sullivan said that interaction was not observed in the small pilot study, but other evidence suggests that both children and adults with ADHD are more at risk for obesity.

Sullivan was also asked to comment on the harmonization of measures or other common elements in related major projects that are under way, such as the Environmental Influences on Child Health Outcomes (ECHO) studies, the Healthy Brain Initiative, and the Healthy Brain and Child Development studies. She said that her group is working with ECHO investigators to try to align their efforts toward common inflammatory and imaging measures in order to expand the sample size, bring more diversity to the study populations, and validate similar measures across sites. Damien Fair, associate professor of behavioral neuroscience, associate professor of psychiatry, and associate scientist at the Advanced Imaging Research Center at the Oregon Health & Science University, added that across those three major projects, researchers are attempting to coordinate brain imaging measurement and processing. Akil remarked that coordinating and standardizing measurements for better reliability as well as validity and cross-comparisons will be important moving forward.

## INSULIN RESISTANCE: A LINK IN BRAIN–BODY INTERACTIONS

In her presentation, Rasgon described how insulin resistance is a link in brain–body interactions. She described the purpose of using insulin as one of the linking agents—both peripherally and centrally—in body and brain connections and explored a conceptual framework for understanding brain health versus brain disease.

### Insulin Resistance and the Link Between Metabolic Dysfunction and Brain Diseases

About 19 years ago, a specific link was postulated between metabolic dysfunction and brain diseases such as affective disorders, mood disorders, and Alzheimer's disease. This metabolic dysfunction was manifested behaviorally through cognitive impairment, giving rise to the idea that the cognitive impairment may be in part attributable to metabolic dysfunction underpinned by the effect of impaired glucose utilization in the brain. As illustrated in Figure 3-4, the multiple mediators and neurotransmitters involved include serotonin and melatonin as part of the serotonin cascade as well as cortisol and estrogen (McIntyre et al., 2009; Rasgon and Jarvik, 2004). The latter is a pivotal hormone responsible for the sex-specific differences in various illnesses, both of the brain and of the body. In this context, the brain–body link relates to the notion of insulin resistance.

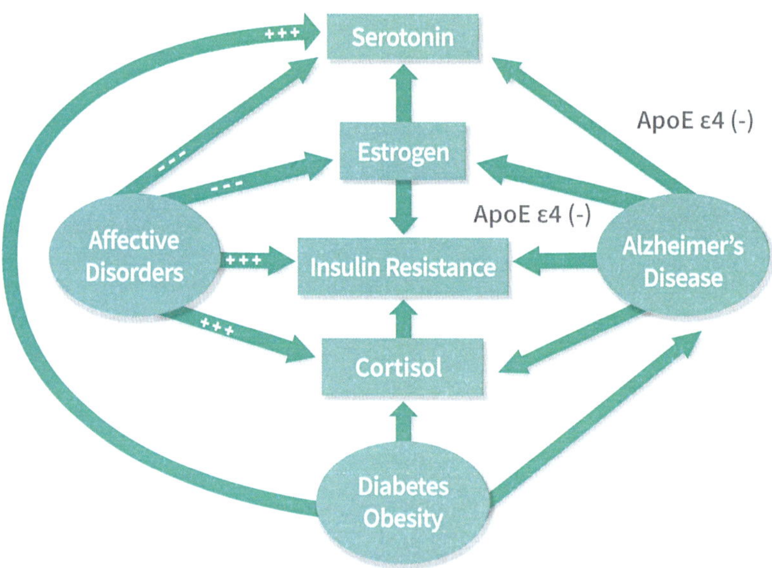


**FIGURE 3-4** Possible mediators of metabolic disruption.
NOTES: Apolipoprotein E (ApoE) is a protein involved in metabolism of fats in the body and highly implicated in the development of Alzheimer's and cardiovascular diseases. ϵ4 is a particular allele of the gene that produces apolipoprotein E, and is the allele most associated with the development of dementia.
SOURCES: As presented by Natalie Rasgon at the workshop Brain Health Across the Life Span on September 24, 2019; adapted from Rasgon and McEwen, 2016.

Rasgon discussed the extent to which insulin resistance may be responsible for the brain–body miscommunication and how it could potentially be used as a target for intervention. The functional effects of insulin have been well established. In the periphery, insulin is specifically responsible for glucose use; in the brain, insulin has a significant adaptive plasticity role and a neuroprotective role. The pleiotropic and pleomorphic representation of the function of insulin makes it an interesting agent to consider as a link between brain and body disorders. Insulin resistance is a condition in which tissue responsiveness to the normal action of insulin is impaired, which may or may not be a consequence of weight gain. It is manifested by decreased insulin receptor sensitivity to the circulating levels of insulin, which can eventually lead to hyperglycemia. Insulin resistance forms a mechanistic foundation for a number of illnesses (Rasgon and Jarvik, 2004; Rasgon et al., 2002). The duration of the lack of tissue responsiveness to insulin and, therefore, the condition of insulin resistance, can last for decades. It does not necessarily result in diabetes in all cases, but it may lead independently to cardiovascular disease, mood disorders, and dementia. In the periphery, the metabolic dysfunction of insulin resistance has distinct endpoints in somatic illness and in central nervous system (CNS) illnesses, including obesity, depression, hypertension, metabolic syndrome, atherosclerosis, diabetes mellitus, microalbuminuria, endothelial dysfunction, and polycystic ovary syndrome.

*Insulin Resistance and Changes in Hippocampal Structure and Function*

Rasgon presented data on insulin resistance and changes in hippocampal structure and function to illustrate how peripheral insulin resistance has correlates in the brain. A number of brain imaging studies have been carried out in subjects aged 45–65 years who were at genetic risk for Alzheimer's disease but did not yet have any identifiable appreciable cognitive impairment. The studies show (1) a direct linear correlation between decreased hippocampal volume and increased insulin resistance in the periphery; (2) decreased connectivity between the hippocampus and prefrontal cortex as insulin resistance increases; and (3) very distinct metabolism impairment in the medial prefrontal cortex attributable to ensuing insulin resistance, according to fluorodeoxyglucose-positron emission tomography (Kenna et al., 2013; Rasgon et al., 2011, 2014). Taken together, these methods for assessing brain correlates of peripheral insulin resistance suggest that there is actually a CNS representation.

### Treating Insulin Resistance in Patients with Mood Disorders

Next, Rasgon considered the "chicken and egg" scenario in the relationship between insulin resistance and mood disorders: which precedes the other, and what can be achieved by modifying peripheral insulin resistance?

#### *Epigenetic Modulation of Metabolic Subtypes of Depression*

Rasgon described a study that found a link between insulin resistance and telomere length in antidepressant response to a peroxisome proliferator-activated receptor gamma (PPARG) agonist, suggesting that there are different metabolic subtypes of depression (Lin et al., 2015). The study looked at the effects of the PPARG agonist pioglitazone, which is an antidiabetic drug used in a placebo-controlled design as adjuvant treatment in patients with unremitted major depression. The subjects' usual treatment for depression was supplemented with pioglitazone or placebo for 3 months. In addition to finding that pioglitazone was effective in reducing depression versus placebo, investigators were able to identify a number of predictors of that treatment response, some of which were specifically related to peripheral insulin resistance. Improvement in depression associated with improvement in glucose metabolism in insulin-resistant subjects and response to pioglitazone was stronger in younger patients. Subjects with longer telomeres, which are known biomarkers of inflammation and allostatic load, exhibited greater declines in depression severity in the active arm, but not in the placebo arm. Based on these data, the investigators posited that there is a metabolic subtype of depression in which depressive disorder is associated with a distinct metabolic signature in the periphery. Furthermore, people with this metabolic subtype may have a different biology and response to treatment with medications typically used for diabetes.

The pioglitazone study spurred further investigation into the epigenetic modulation of the metabolic subtype of depression. Work by the National Institute on Aging (NIA) reversibility research network on the effect of early childhood adversity on cognitive performance in midlife has revealed that early childhood adversity is a pivotal moment—it is both a window of vulnerability and a window of opportunity. In looking at biological processes, there is evidence that emotional abuse is associated with multiple biological and neurobiological correlates to depression. A number of biomarkers of allostatic load and stress are predicted by childhood trauma and are related to peripheral insulin resistance. This allows for deeper endophenotyping of the metabolic type of depression: it is associated with childhood trauma, it is insulin resistant in the periphery, and it is manifested by multiple distinct molecules as predictors of decreased emotion regulation and cognitive regulation in the brain (Bigio et al., 2016; Nasca et al., 2018). One of those molecules is acetylcarnitine, an epigenetic glutamatergic modulator, which has subsequent downstream effects in the brain.

### *Novel Mechanisms of Brain Plasticity in Mood and Cognition*

Work on acetylcarnitine indicates that in the cross talk between the brain and the body, deficient plasticity has a significant number of mediators, said Rasgon. Although it is not yet clear which mediators precede the others, the data suggest that the combination of sex differences driven by estrogen that make women more vulnerable to childhood trauma is compounded by subsequent metabolic dysfunction, in which glutamatergic changes can trigger the cascade of changes in neuronal plasticity (Nasca et al., 2017). It is already understood how these peripheral events and central events collate because of our understanding of diabetes prevalence and comorbidities and multimorbidities between the various illnesses represented by these deficiencies.

Studies of acetylcarnitine deficiency in subjects with major depressive disorder and treatment-resistant depression have also illustrated the changes in the glutamatergic modulator system in the brains of those patients. Compared to healthy controls, the patients with severe depression have a nearly linear decline in glutamatergic plasticity (Nasca et al., 2018). This same agent is also a mediator of insulin resistance—this time in the brain. Looking at central insulin resistance reveals that there could potentially be cross talk between the body and the brain in the molecular signature of those regulatory factors, but it could also be two completely distinct processes unrelated to each other. Data are emerging from studies of in vivo brain insulin resistance in patients with major depressive disorder and characterized by acetylcarnitine deficiency, suggesting that there is an in vivo nanotechnology method that can be used to assess actual central insulin resistance by measuring the same biomarkers of insulin function among others in exosomes, which are the peripherally circulating baggage from the central nervous system. By enriching for the brain-derived exosomes and looking at the specific insulin receptor substrate concentration in those brain-derived exosomes, investigators are finding that healthy controls have significantly less turnover of the insulin-resistant substrate.[5]

[5] Rasgon, N. Workshop PowerPoint presentation—Insulin Resistance: A Link in Brain–Body Interactions. Available at http://www.nationalacademies.org/hmd/Activities/Aging/BrainHealthAcrossTheLifeSpanWorkshop/2019-JUN-26.aspx (accessed March 12, 2020).

### Future Research Directions

Rasgon concluded by outlining future directions based on the findings of the mechanistic studies she described. Figure 3-5 illustrates potential trajectories over the life span from health to risk, then to poor health and disease. Early-life adversity can be associated with metabolic phenotypes, with future studies needed to further elucidate the biochemical pathways involved and to identify potential targets for intervention. This conceptualization situates pregnancy-related metabolic and psychological events as the starting points that can trigger trajectories at different stages, which are mediated along the way by a range of normal and pathological, environmental, and internal conditions. The trajectories begin with convergence at early life but then diverge with various life events.

Rasgon highlighted the factors of allostatic load and resilience as main points of interest for trying to identify important milestones and windows for intervention. She added that within this framework of bilateral communication, reverse translation is as important as direct translation.

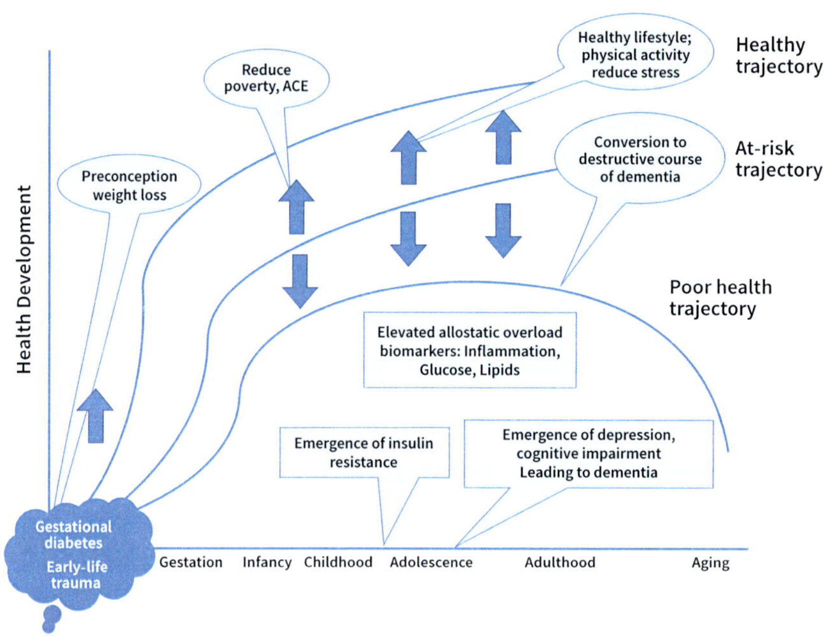


**FIGURE 3-5** Potential trajectories of health over the life span.
NOTE: ACE = adverse childhood experience.
SOURCES: As presented by Natalie Rasgon at the workshop Brain Health Across the Life Span on September 24, 2019; Watson et al., 2018.

Therefore, an important future research direction is to identify phenotypic presentations in cohorts of people with illness, then to return to animal studies to try to understand mechanisms that underlie those presentations. This would allow for testing potential interventions in large cohorts. This should also include multifaceted interventions that involve not only the biological interventions but also various psychosocial strategies for augmenting and improving the delivery of those biological interventions.

## Discussion

Rasgon was asked to elaborate on the correlation between insulin resistance, corticoids, and other component factors of stress. She explained that insulin receptors are highly collinear with the cortisol receptors in the hippocampus. They are expressed in the same regions, and they have a mutually potentiating effect of insulin and cortisol toxicity. Models of major depression, for example, show that people with major depression have an overproduction of cortisol and increased insulin resistance in the brain, specifically in the hippocampus. The same also holds in the periphery, she said. People with Cushing's syndrome, for instance, have primary hypercortisolemia, which is a well-known model for insulin resistance and for mood disorder, so there is a strong correlation between them. Stress as a concept is a very multinomial construct, she added. Studies tend to focus only on stress that leads to negative outcomes, with the notion of positive stress often overlooked in research. She suggested that this is a research gap to be addressed—perhaps it may be even more stressful to have a healthy brain and joyful experience. She surmised that positive stress could have a bigger imprint in the brain than having a negative effect, because people may be more used to dealing with adversity than to dealing with joy.

Lis Nielsen, chief of the Individual Behavioral Processes Branch of the Division of Behavioral and Social Research at NIA, asked about potential nonpharmacological lifestyle interventions along the insulin resistance pathway. Rasgon said that work is ongoing in both humans and animals. New animal data are emerging on the transmission of behavioral and biological imprints from biological mothers to offspring. This epigenetic modulation relates not only to trauma and upbringing but also relates to diet and to the level and extent of physical activity (not necessarily rigorous and nonrigorous exercise). Because these factors contribute to pathophysiology, interventions that target food intake, food composition, and caloric intake could have a positive effect related to the effect of insulin resistance on the metabolic endophenotype of depression and subsequent cognitive diseases. Going forward, research efforts should focus on a combination of psychopharmacological, behavioral, and environmental interventions, Rasgon said.

## PANEL DISCUSSION ON BRAIN–BODY INTERACTIONS

To begin the discussion, Bruce McEwen, Alfred E. Mirsky Professor at The Rockefeller University, commented on the positive functions of circadian rhythms and metabolic hormones. Ultradian (rhythms longer than 1 hour but less than 1 day) and circadian variation of cortisol facilitate the turnover of synapses in many parts of the brain, enabling motor learning. If the circadian variation is disrupted and cortisol is elevated at the wrong time, or disturbs the sleep–wake cycle, then these effects are impaired such that the brain is not able to adapt as efficiently. In the context of metabolic hormones, McEwen noted the idea that the insulin-like growth factor 1 (IGF1) hormone from the liver is required for exercise to stimulate neurogenesis in the dentate gyrus of the hippocampus; if IGF1 is blocked in animal studies, exercise no longer stimulates neurogenesis. In fact, a number of other hormonal factors from muscle and bone, and perhaps other parts of the body, also facilitate this and other processes of plasticity. Another surprising facet of metabolic hormones is that both lectin and growth hormone are made in the brain, especially in the hippocampus, but they can also come from outside the brain and have complementary effects for neuroprotection to enhance cognitive and other functions. The same is true for prolactin and ghrelin; hippocampal studies show that they do not appear to be made in the brain, but they can access the brain and have generally neuroprotective effects. However, problems occur when the brain becomes resistant to those hormones.

### Need for Basic Neuroscience to Adopt a Holistic Perspective

Akil remarked that basic neuroscientists should focus on nonneuronal cell types and take a more holistic perspective on the brain as part of the entire body—meaning, thinking also about the ways in which the brain is a target of the body, rather than thinking about neurocircuitry and the brain in isolation. She noted that a question that commonly arises in discussions about the burden of brain disorders is whether the apparent increase in prevalence of disorders such as autism and Alzheimer's disease is attributable to people's brains becoming less healthy or to an increase in the willingness to talk about, diagnose, and report brain disorders. Similarly, brain disorders related to aging are often framed as an inevitable consequence of people living to older ages, without sufficient consideration as to how brain health is influenced by a person's body, their eating and sleeping habits, fulfillment of their basic needs, and how the person interacts with the external physical world.

## Continuum of Brain Health and Disease

To help clarify where health ends and disease begins, said Rasgon, a continuum may be more useful than a more parsimonious illness-versus-health construct. Unlike infectious diseases, brain disorders and somatic disorders such as diabetes have lengthy and continuing effects; for example, prediabetes can last for decades before it becomes diabetes; cognitive impairment can precede dementia but may never get to the end stage. Brain diseases—as with many "body" diseases—are not discrete events in time. They may develop as a continuum and accumulation, mirroring the relationship between stress and allostatic load. It is now understood that neurodegeneration can begin very early in life. If neonates and children have genetic risk factor APOE4 for Alzheimer's disease, they tend to have smaller hippocampi. Although this does not mean they will necessarily get Alzheimer's disease, they already have certain changes in the brain. This underscores the difficulty in drawing a distinct line between what constitutes illness versus health.

Akil agreed about the need to shift the perspective away from the cause-and-cure binary. She added that the field of medicine more broadly is often biased toward focusing on conditions such as infections or injuries that have clear triggers, treatments, and endpoints. This is evident in early global health efforts that focused on infectious diseases. Similarly, in the field of genetics, there is a tendency to identify a single faulty gene as the source of the problem. However, probabilistic thinking then shifts bias and risk over a longer time frame, which reveals cumulative effects. Many brain disorders have patterns that are not discrete—they are slower, longer, and cumulative, which gives rise to questions about how to measure the disorder and the boundaries of the potential windows for intervention (e.g., when is too early, when is too late).

A participant noted that a state of balance can be attained after a brain disorder diagnosis such as obsessive–compulsive disorder (OCD) or bipolar disorder, for example, and asked if a person in that state of balance would not experience symptoms. Rasgon said that OCD and bipolar disorder are treatable, but not curable; other brain disorders such as Alzheimer's disease are not yet even treatable. Although it is possible to contain the presentation of these types of illnesses, it does not mean that the illness is gone. McClung added that there is no consensus about the starting point of bipolar disorder. Some people believe that it occurs after a discrete break during adolescence—meaning, there is no childhood bipolar disorder. Others believe that the disorder begins much earlier and that certain factors can predict which children are at risk of developing the full-blown disease. Circadian rhythm patterns of the sleep–wake cycle in children can predict worse outcomes in terms of bipolar disorder and schizophrenia. Researchers are also looking at sleep patterns related to schizophrenia. For example, people with schizophrenia have disease-specific disrupted sleep spindles that also occur prepsychosis in at-risk subjects. She agreed that the field of brain health seems to be shifting its focus to understanding the early stages of diseases, noting that early intervention to try to prevent diseases is a better strategy than trying to treat them once they have progressed.

Akil suggested that some brain disorders do not have a discrete beginning and ending. If a person with a seizure disorder, for example, receives the optimal combination of treatments and has not had a seizure for decades, then that person has a higher risk of seizure, but has achieved a state of health in general. Furthermore, the seeds of brain disorders are multifactorial, spanning the biology of the brain, genetics, maternal context, and the early-life uterine environment, but also a host of other factors and life events that are less understood but contribute to the manifestation of a disorder. She added that a brain disorder itself is another important agent—for instance, being bipolar is itself a stressor and a burden—which contributes to a vicious cycle. Breaking those cycles is an important part of resetting the trajectory of illness.

### Toward a Preventive, Life-Course Approach to Brain Health

Discussing brain health in the context of disease is an appropriate starting point, said Nielsen. However, decisions about how to define the presence of disease can be avoided by moving toward a preventive, long-term, life-course perspective about avoiding disease through resilience, restorative processes, and the potential to achieve positive health by mitigating risk factors or early exposures. Rasgon said that preventive interventions should focus on implementing education and behavioral paradigms where they are needed the most, such as underserved populations and communities with limited access to health care.

Researchers in the field are consistently finding that familial transmission and upbringing are dimensions in which education can modify potential risk and potentially limit children's exposure to vulnerabilities that lead to risk factors for disease. Educating parents who are living with an illness about how their own lifestyles are modeled by their children—both positively and negatively—could help to identify earlier windows of opportunity for interventions to ensure that the next generation does not become a vulnerable group as well. Akil remarked that relatively simple public health interventions related to lifestyle factors (e.g., diet, sleep, exercise) that promote general health are the foundation of brain health (NRC and IOM, 2000). McEwen pointed out that in terms of interventions, one size does not fit all. It is important to look at a person's early-life history to identify windows of opportunity for change at different periods in time, not only during infancy and childhood but also extending into adolescence and young adulthood (NASEM, 2019).

Rasgon offered a vignette based on the clear transmission of the risk for ADHD with a high-fat diet. She suggested that if having ADHD and obesity negatively affects a person's parenting style, then some children of those parents may respond to emotional distress by self-medicating with unhealthy food. This in itself is a primary preceding metabolic dysfunction that may lead to brain illness. Because it is already widely understood that somatic illnesses such as obesity are detrimental to overall health, she suggested that a simple way to operationalize this complexity in public messaging is to highlight the brain health outcomes of those illnesses as well as their physical health outcomes.

McClung commented that an opportunity for change is to dispel widespread misperceptions about the amount of sleep that children and adolescents actually need and about the consequences of sleep deprivation. Typical school start times are a directly modifiable factor that would benefit adolescents broadly, but especially among those at risk. Children or adolescents with a family history of psychiatric disease should be on a preventive schedule that allows them to have the appropriate amount of sleep within a structured circadian cycle. Advocacy efforts are already under way to push back school start times, but they are generally met with resistance.

### Measurement Strategies

Akil highlighted the task of defining what needs to be measured. McClung described how measuring circadian rhythms can be used to predict "crashes" in people with bipolar or other disorders in which circadian rhythmicity is part of the symptomatology, as well as how measuring rhythm can be used to administer drugs at the appropriate time. Rasgon discussed how measurement can be used to distinguish between different types of depression to determine whether regular antidepressant treatment should be augmented with anti-insulin resistance treatment in certain people. Simple early childhood measurements can also be used to predict the child's risk of developing ADHD later on in life. She asked participants to discuss the extent to which whether measuring physiological markers such as circadian rhythm, metabolic levels, and insulin resistance is truly relevant to brain health, or whether they are just low-hanging fruit. Nielsen replied that the NIH Science of Behavior Change initiative is concentrating on promoting brain health by persuading people to adopt and maintain lifelong healthy behavioral patterns—with adherence to those patterns being the linchpin. Work in the field of behavior change is focused on identifying and tailoring interventions to specific malleable psychological and behavioral targets, but the challenge ahead will be to address the behavioral phenotypes that characterize people's amenability to various forms of intervention, such as public health messaging, in order to effect real long-term changes in people's lifestyles. For instance, some people may need specific assessment of their behavioral plasticity and ability to be intervened upon—captured via some psychological or psychobiological measure—that will provide guidance about how to intervene and support maintenance and adherence.

McClung pointed out several studies that could be instructive about how measurements can be used to determine the optimal type of treatment for a patient, rather than relying on the trial-and-error approach common in current psychiatric practice. Studies on both depression and bipolar disorder have used measurements to predict treatment response. One study used actigraphy watches in people with depression to measure their circadian rhythms over a period of time, before receiving an acute dose of ketamine. Investigators were able to predict which people responded to treatment based on their previous circadian rhythms and—because ketamine enhances circadian rhythms in certain people—they were able to predict the people in which ketamine would have a lasting effect. Studies have also found that although people with bipolar disorder all have circadian rhythms that are disrupted, some have longer rhythms, and some have shorter. People who have a shorter rhythm respond better to lithium, because lithium lengthens the rhythm, while people who have a longer rhythm respond better to valproic acid.

Akil asked how to ensure that this type of knowledge can be translated more broadly into actions that can empower people who want to achieve greater health. As huge amounts of data become available at our fingertips from actigraphy and other rapid, easy measurements, it will likely become clear that some people benefit from ongoing feedback about their own data and use it to drive improvement in behavior, while other people may be much less interested. The field of brain health should seek to provide tools that match a range of styles and personalities, which will require another level of analysis. In addition to providing people with their own data, social supports will be needed to inform preventive measures and promote healthier lifestyles.

# 4

# Behavioral and Biological Convergence

**Key Points Highlighted by Workshop Participants**

- The concept of brain health involves our ability to safely and successfully navigate the world around us, and attention is a major cognitive process underpinning this ability. (Monica Rosenberg)
- From a research perspective, predictive modeling approaches will help to move functional magnetic resonance imaging from a science of group averages—meaning, elucidating what happens in the brain on average when people pay attention—toward a science of individual differences. (Monica Rosenberg)
- Going forward in research, it will be important to characterize the brain signatures of different types of attention without assuming that "more is always better." (Monica Rosenberg)
- The concept of resilience refers to the ability of most people, when exposed even to extraordinary levels of stress and trauma, to maintain normal psychological and physical functioning and avoid serious mental illness. (Elizabeth Hoge)
- Several strategies can be used to measure resilience in humans: (1) examining people who have experienced adversity, stress, or trauma and then function well later; (2) bringing

people into the laboratory, stressing them, and then measuring their ability to cope; or (3) administering self-report questionnaires. The third strategy is the most commonly used to measure resilience in the available literature. There is a need to move the field toward validating these commonly used pencil-and-paper measures against some kind of behavioral measures. (Elizabeth Hoge)

- In the context of defining resilience, it is important to consider how long a negative reaction persists; the memory of positive versus negative experiences could be used as one potential measure of resilience. (Huda Akil)
- Resilience relates to the capacity to cope with stress. A person experiencing bad stress may feel overwhelmed and lacking in the resources to cope, while a person experiencing good stress believes they have the resources to cope with it. Resilience could thus be defined by a person's belief in his or her ability to cope and succeed in the face of stress without negative mental or physical health outcomes. Within this paradigm, it could be useful to help people transform bad stress into good stress, so they feel more confident and capable without being preoccupied by their past mistakes. (Elizabeth Hoge)
- Resilience is a concept best thought of over time, because it seems to involve dynamic processing to "bounce back" after a challenging situation. (Monica Rosenberg)
- It is likely that the brain has multiple capacities and systems that are related to resilience. Striving for a single unifying definition of resilience—in the service of identifying specific measurable psychological capacities—could occlude the idea that resilience constitutes multiple capacities that interact with each other. (Lis Nielsen)
- The most difficult step in research on the brain and cognitive processes related to resilience is to identify whether a given brain phenomenon is a risk factor or a response. Differentiating between the two, while challenging, is critical for characterizing the brain's response to stress and how to manage it to improve long-term outcomes. (Damien Fair)
- From a research perspective, it is useful to consider the potential distinction between emotional and cognitive resilience. Cognitive resilience could be described as a system that is perturbed by some life event, but the system is still able to function on a longer time scale. In other words, cognitive

resilience amounts to neurodegeneration that does not result in a major collapse of cognitive abilities, as opposed to organic damage of some kind. (Gagan Wig)

- Because of the difficulty in defining concepts of resilience, stress, and brain health, multimodal measures are important, such as measuring self-reported emotion over time in addition to adrenocorticotropic hormone or cortisol levels in the brain. (Lis Nielsen)

This chapter focuses on behavioral and biological convergence in brain health. Presenters and panelists discussed the connections and discontinuities between brain activity and behavior as well as those between psychological health and brain health. They examined what behavior and life experience may suggest about brain health and resilience. The biological underpinnings of behavior in the context of cognition, emotion, and psychiatric disorders were also explored. Monica Rosenberg, assistant professor in the department of psychology at the University of Chicago, provided an overview of the neural correlates of attention and cognition. Elizabeth Hoge, director of the anxiety disorders research program at the Georgetown University Medical Center, considered the question of whether meditation can improve health and resilience.

## NEURAL CORRELATES OF ATTENTION AND COGNITION

Rosenberg explored the neural correlates of attention and cognition by describing how attentional and cognitive processes can be characterized using predictive models based on brain data. She described the concept of brain health as generally involving our ability to safely and successfully navigate the world around us. Attention is a major cognitive process that is the cornerstone of the brain's executive functions. It is important for life outcomes across development (e.g., children who pay better attention have better educational outcomes during their school years). However, the ability to pay attention varies across different people; the ability also varies in the same person over time. Attention lapses are common but can have negative consequences, as illustrated by the spike in car accidents in recent years caused by drivers who were distracted by their phones. Her presentation focused on how brain-based models can be used to predict attentional abilities, to capture changes in attention over time, and to characterize individual differences in working memory during development.

## Functional Brain Connectivity

Many psychological tasks, questionnaires, and clinical measures can be used to measure differences in attention between people and within people. Rosenberg proposed that brain measures can be used to complement these behavioral measures of attention, focusing on the role of functional brain connectivity as a useful brain measure. Functional brain connectivity can be assessed through a functional magnetic resonance imaging (fMRI) scan of the brain. Based on the scan, brain activity is divided into several hundred regions or nodes. Researchers can then look at the activity signal time course in one node and correlate it with a single time course in every other node, generating a whole-brain connectivity matrix or connectome. In the matrix shown in Figure 4-1, the rows and columns represent distinct brain regions; cells represent the correlation between activity in those regions. The matrix can then be projected back onto the brain. Rosenberg explained that the lines in between the nodes are statistical interactions—specifically, they are correlation coefficients—that do not necessarily represent structural connections between brain regions.

Functional connectivity is the measure being focused on because evidence suggests that every person has a unique pattern of functional brain connectivity, a "functional connectivity fingerprint," that is relatively stable over time and contains information about cognitive abilities (Finn et al., 2015; Miranda-Dominguez et al., 2014), including fluid intelligence, which can be used to predict attention and other abilities. She emphasized that more broadly, these types of predictive modeling approaches will help to move fMRI from a science of group averages—meaning, elucidating what happens in the brain on average when people pay attention—toward a science of individual differences. This could potentially enable a single brain scan to provide specific information about an individual person's brain, abilities, outcomes, and most appropriate treatments or

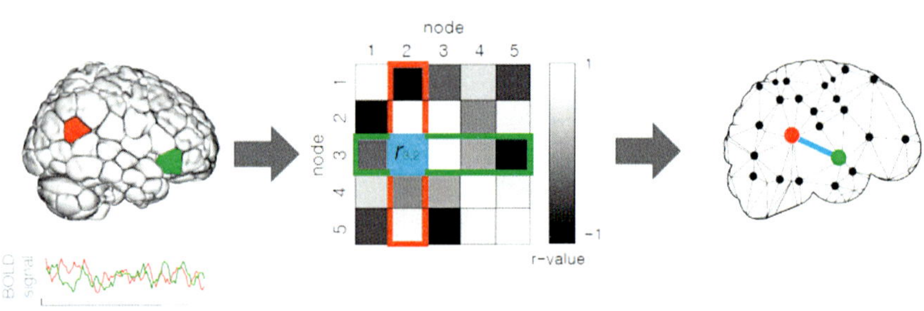


**FIGURE 4-1** Measuring functional brain connectivity.
SOURCE: Adapted from figures presented by Monica Rosenberg at the workshop Brain Health Across the Life Span on September 24, 2019.

interventions. However, care must be taken to test model generalizability, to control for confounds, and to ensure that predictions are robust and meaningful.

### Use of Brain-Based Models to Predict Attentional Abilities

Rosenberg described some of her laboratory's work in using brain-based models to predict attentional abilities (Shen et al., 2017). Connectome-based predictive modeling was used to capture individual differences in sustained attention in adulthood and to capture real-world attention-deficit hyperactivity disorder (ADHD) symptoms in a cognitively developing population (Rosenberg et al., 2016a). An overview of the process of connectome-based predictive modeling is provided in Box 4-1.

**BOX 4-1**
**Connectome-Based Predictive Modeling**

The first step in connectome-based predictive modeling is to identify which of the tens of thousands of functional connections in the whole-brain pattern are related to the behavioral measure of interest. To do so, investigators leave out data from a single subject and correlate the strength of every connection with behavior across the remaining subjects, generating a matrix that indicates the relationship between the strength of a functional connection and behavior across individuals. Researchers then retain the connections that are most strongly related to behavior in the positive and the negative directions. For instance, a high-attention network would include the set of functional connections that are stronger in people who are performing well on the task; the low-attention network would include the set of connections that are stronger in people who are performing poorly. Neither network contains functional connections or correlation coefficients that are exclusively positive or negative—they are simply positively or negatively related to behavior.

Rosenberg emphasized that everybody expresses both of these networks, but they are expressed to a different degree in each person. The next step in the approach is to formally relate strength to behavior in these networks using a linear model. This is carried out by looking at the degree to which each participant expresses the network overall—by summing up the functional connection strengths in the network—and relating that to behavior. Models are validated by applying them to data from previously unseen individuals to generate behavioral predictions.

SOURCE: As presented by Monica Rosenberg at the workshop Brain Health Across the Life Span on September 24, 2019.

*Capturing Individual Differences in Sustained Attention in Adults*

To operationalize individual differences in sustained attention in adults, the researchers used a gradual-onset continuous performance task (Esterman et al., 2013). Brain imaging data were collected from 25 healthy adults while they were performing a challenging task requiring continuous, sustained attention. In addition to measures of whole-brain functional connectivity, task performance was also measured for each subject. The aim was to use the functional connectivity patterns to predict task performance using connectome-based predictive modeling (Rosenberg et al., 2016a; Shen et al., 2017).[1]

In this case, the expected effect would be that people who express the high-attention network more strongly overall would perform better on the task, while people who express the low-attention network more strongly would perform worse. The analysis procedure guarantees that the features are actually predicting attention, and they are not simply related to the selected measure by chance. Specifically, the investigators leave out data from a single subject and correlate the strength of every connection with behavior across the remaining subjects, generating a matrix that indicates the relationship between the strength of a functional connection and behavior across individuals. Data from the left-out person are then brought back into the model to see how strongly the person expressed the networks. This measure is used to predict how well the left-out person performed on the task. Iterating this process through all of the subjects—leaving each person out once—allows for a predicted measure of performance for each individual to be derived. Thus, how people actually performed on the task can be plotted against how they were predicted to perform, based on their connectivity patterns.

When Rosenberg's group made predictions using the high-attention network model, they captured a significant variance in performance—more than 70 percent of the variance—in how people perform the task, based on brain data alone (Rosenberg et al., 2016a). They achieved similar performance when making predictions with the low-attention network model as well as a model that takes into account strength in both networks.[2] Next, her group applied the models to data collected while participants were just resting in the scanner and not doing any task. The aim was to compare these rest predictions with the task predictions to determine whether subjects needed to perform an attention task at all in order for researchers to predict how well they pay attention, as well as

[1] The code associated with this technique, visualization tools, and a detailed protocol are available online at github.com/YaleMRRC/CPM (accessed November 3, 2019).

[2] They are now exploring the possibility that the high- and low-attention network models may be providing some degree of redundant information.

whether the functional architecture of attention is reflected in the brain while a person is lying in the scanner looking at a fixation cross on the screen. Rest data were also able to predict performance.

Although the predictions were not as accurate as those based on task data, her team was still able to explain significant variants in participants' performance based only on their functional connectivity patterns observed at rest. Figure 4-2 depicts plots of the prediction from task data and from rest data. Rosenberg suggested that task predictions are better than the rest predictions because engaging in the attention task perturbs circuits relevant to sustained attention, potentially magnifying these behaviorally relevant individual differences. She likened psychological tasks to "stress tests" for certain types of processes like attention (Finn et al., 2017).

### *Predicting Attention-Deficit Hyperactivity Disorder Symptoms in Children and Adolescents*

To capture a broader concept of sustained attention, rather than focusing on predicting performance on an idiosyncratic lab-based task, the researchers applied the model to data collected in a very different

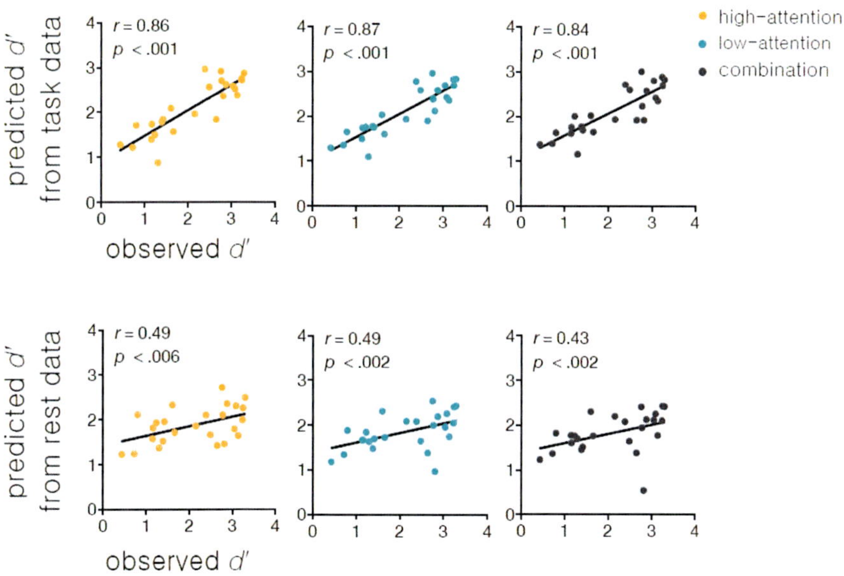


**FIGURE 4-2** Predicting task performance based on functional connectivity patterns.
SOURCES: As presented by Monica Rosenberg at the workshop Brain Health Across the Life Span on September 24, 2019; Rosenberg et al., 2016a.

context—publicly available data[3] from children and adolescents with ADHD.[4] For each child, there was a resting-state functional connectivity pattern and a measure of ADHD symptoms rated by clinicians using the ADHD Rating Scale IV. Rosenberg noted that her group had scores for children that had received an ADHD diagnosis, as well as for children who did not have a diagnosis, so they were predicting continuous measures of symptom severity in both patients and controls.

The goal of this analysis was to apply the model to predict how each child or adolescent would perform if (hypothetically) given the same continuous performance task that the adults received in the laboratory (Rosenberg et al., 2017). The expected negative result emerged when Rosenberg's group plotted the severity of ADHD symptoms on the x-axis (with higher scores indicating more frequent or more severe symptoms) and predicted task performance on the y-axis. When they predicted that a child or adolescent would perform well on the task, the subject showed fewer symptoms or less severe symptoms of ADHD. This suggests that the model is capturing something in general about the ability to sustain attention, not just something specific about performance on one laboratory-based task.

To assess whether the model was specifically predicting abilities related to attention as opposed to, for example, predicting the ability to comply with instruction and to be high functioning overall, her team analyzed whether the predictions were related to ADHD scores when controlling for intelligence quotient (IQ); the predictions were not related to IQ scores when controlling for ADHD scores. These predictions are general, in that they are generalizing across datasets and across measures of sustained attention and across age groups. However, the predictions are also specific, in that they are predicting scores specifically related to attention.

### *High- and Low-Attention Network Anatomies*

Rosenberg explained that data-driven predictive approaches can inform the functional architecture of attention and cognition. Specifically, she presented data to illustrate the anatomy of high- and low-attention data-driven networks in the brain (Rosenberg et al., 2016a, 2017). In summary, she showed that brain regions (or nodes) can be characterized by how many connections they have in both high- and low-attention networks, and the proportion of connections in each. Together, these connections

---

[3] The ADHD-200 Sample: http://fcon_1000.projects.nitrc.org/indi/adhd200 (accessed February 3, 2020).

[4] From the ADHD 200 dataset and data collected in China from 113 children and adolescents aged 8–13 years.

in high- and low-attention networks only represent about 4 percent of all possible functional connections in the networks. Some nodes are highly specialized in one network or the other, whereas other nodes have approximately equal numbers of connections in the network predicting better attention and the network predicting worse attention. She emphasized that when predicting differences in attention, the functional connectivity measure is particularly important—it is not the individual brain regions per se that matter, but rather the statistical interactions between the activity time courses of pairs of brain regions.

Data-driven techniques like this one can serve as hypothesis generators by suggesting regions or connections that were not previously known to be related to attention. They can also confirm previous hypotheses or agree with work in the field. For example, one feature of the low-attention network is the large number of functional connections between hemispheres of the cerebellum. This agrees with work in ADHD suggesting that cerebellar changes are particularly relevant.

## Using Brain-Based Models to Capture Changes in Attention Over Time

Rosenberg turned to the use of brain-based models to capture changes in attention over time. If her laboratory's model is related to the ability to focus, it should also change with attentional changes over time. Emerging evidence suggests that some connectome-based models are capturing changes in attention within a single person; this has been documented and suggested in the literature (Adam et al., 2015, 2018; Christoff et al., 2009; Cohen and Maunsell, 2011; deBettencourt et al., 2018; Esterman et al., 2013; Rosenberg et al., 2013; Sali et al., 2016; Smilek et al., 2010). To determine whether their model was sensitive to changes in attention over time, her team measured the same person doing the same continuous attention task while being scanned by fMRI at 30 different time points over 11 months (Salehi et al., 2020). This yielded a functional connectivity matrix and task performance assessment from each of the 30 sessions. The task performance at each session was plotted against the model's prediction of the subject's performance based on connectivity in every session-specific pattern. Rosenberg's group found that the model is sensitive to the individual's daily changes in task performance (Rosenberg et al., 2020). If the model was only sensitive to the person's average attentional ability, no relationships between changes in this connectivity signature of attention and changes in behavior would be expected, but the model was actually sensitive to the person's best session and worst session. It was also very accurate in capturing the person's overall general average sustained attention ability in addition to capturing changes in attention from session to session.

*Use of Brain-Based Models to Capture Changes in Attention Caused by Pharmacological Interaction*

Rosenberg noted that daily or moment-to-moment fluctuations in attention are commonplace, but attention also changes with pharmacological intervention. She presented data from a study in which healthy adults were given either a single dose of methylphenidate or no drug at all (Farr et al., 2014a,b; Rosenberg et al., 2016b). Methylphenidate is a common ADHD treatment that blocks dopamine and/or epinephrine reuptake (Berridge et al., 2006; Spencer et al., 2015; Volkow et al., 2001). It is very effective, providing symptom improvement in about 70 percent of patients with ADHD (Greenhill et al., 2002); performance enhancements are also seen even in participants who are not diagnosed with ADHD. Investigators examined high- and low-attention network strength in a group of adults given a single dose of methylphenidate before the scan—as expected, individuals given the attention-enhancing drug showed functional connectivity signatures of better attention. That is, participants who had been administered methylphenidate showed higher high-attention network strength and lower low-attention network strength than control participants who received no medication. This indicates that methylphenidate is not just having an effect on a person's functional connectivity overall; rather, it is selectively modulating the functional connections related to attentional abilities. The same pattern was observed both when people were performing a stop-signal task and when they were simply resting. This set of studies suggests that the same models that predict individual differences in attention are also capturing fluctuations in attention within people over time, as well as changes in attention resulting from pharmacological interventions.

Beyond characterizing individual differences in sustained attention, these functional connectivity patterns and predictive modeling methods can also be used to capture individual differences in a number of different abilities, behaviors, or clinical symptoms (Shen et al., 2017). For instance, these patterns can be used to predict aspects of adult working-memory function (Avery et al., 2020), adult fluid intelligence (Finn et al., 2015), and autism symptoms (Lake et al., 2019). Work is ongoing across many research groups to share and validate functional connectivity biomarkers and evaluate the degree to which they generalize across datasets. "If we really want to move toward an individualized translational neuroscience and applications, we need to confirm that our models generalize beyond the single dataset on which they are built," Rosenberg noted.

## Use of Brain-Based Models to Characterize Working Memory in Development

Rosenberg explained how a different type of brain measure and brain-based predictive model is being used to characterize working memory in developmental periods such as childhood and adolescence. Working memory is a critical cognitive ability related to processing speed, fluid intelligence, and attention that allows a person to store and manipulate information in the mind (Baddeley, 1992; Kane and Engle, 2002). Like attention, working memory varies significantly between individuals and changes across development (Klingberg et al., 2002). Previous work suggests that these differences are supported by frontoparietal circuitry in the brain (Darki and Klingberg, 2015; Klingberg et al., 2002; Palva et al., 2010; Satterthwaite et al., 2013). Mental disorders, including ADHD, anxiety and mood disorders, schizophrenia, and substance abuse, tend to emerge and peak during adolescence (Lee et al., 2014). The ability to predict symptoms and abilities earlier in development (prior to adulthood) could offer greater opportunities to intervene earlier and to afford people improved outcomes.

### *Relationships Between Functional Magnetic Resonance Imaging Activity and Working Memory*

To that end, initiatives like the Adolescent Brain Cognitive Development Study (ABCD) are collecting and sharing large developmental datasets with MRI data, as well as providing resources to train and test predictive models (Rosenberg et al., 2018). Rosenberg described the results of one project that used data from the first release of ABCD data (including more than 5,000 children aged 9–10 years collected at 21 sites across the United States) to characterize individual differences in working memory. Activation in frontoparietal regions during a challenging working-memory task (e.g., a two-back task)[5] relative to a lower-load working-memory task (e.g., a zero-back task), was significantly related to out-of-scanner working-memory performance (Rosenberg et al., 2019). This indicates that children who have stronger working-memory abilities tend to have greater activation in the frontoparietal regions during a working-memory challenge than children with less strong abilities.

Such differences are not seen with brain activation in other contexts, such as activation during emotional versus neutral face blocks of the emotional *n*-back task. Similarly, no differences were observed in data

[5] A task in which participants are presented several stimuli in a row, and then asked to determine whether the current stimulus is the same as a stimulus shown two steps earlier.

collected during an inhibitory control task (stop-signal task) or a reward processing task (monetary incentive delay task). This suggests that 9- and 10-year-olds with stronger working memories do not simply have greater engagement of frontoparietal circuitry overall in any challenging context. Rosenberg reiterated that psychological tasks can be thought of as stress tests for elucidating individual differences in brain activity related to behavior. Brain-related differences are observed in children with stronger and weaker working memories when they are given an explicit working-memory challenge but not in the other contexts tested.

## Discussion

Huda Akil, codirector and research professor of the Molecular and Behavioral Neuroscience Institute and Quarton Professor of Neurosciences at the University of Michigan, asked for clarification about how it was possible to pick up changes in sustained attention over time and with treatment, given the lack of sufficient continuity to make predictions without the person actually doing the task. She also asked whether sustained attention is best conceptualized as a trait, a state, or a combination of both. Rosenberg replied that the analysis shows that it is possible to capture differences from day to day in a single person as well as to capture the person's mean or average of attentional focus in a variety of contexts. Factors like motivation, context, sleep, and caffeine all influence whether the person will achieve the maximum or minimum level of focus that fluctuates around that day-to-day average. The models seem to be picking up that type of average mean ability, but they are also sensitive to changes.

Work is ongoing to collect more data on single individuals, in addition to high-throughput big data samples, which should help to tease apart these state-like versus trait-like effects. Evidence suggests that this functional connectivity fingerprint is relatively stable across development and over time, but it can be altered to some degree by task states, cognitive states, and pharmacological states. Akil added that this raises ethical questions related to publicly available brain signatures.

Martha Snyder Taggart, science writer and staff member at BrightFocus Health, asked Rosenberg if her team had observed any subjects with cross-correlated thinking types, such as creativity, who may have more tendencies to integrate against attention. Rosenberg replied that they have not looked at the relationship between those types of factors and attention, but they have investigated the relationship between functional connectivity in general with personality traits and creativity. Her team found that connectivity patterns predicted people's divergent thinking abilities, which have been generalized across multiple independent datasets collected across various continents. Work from other laboratories has suggested that other patterns predict aspects of personality.

A participant asked if the relationship between circadian rhythms and attention or reaction times has been explored. Rosenberg responded that her lab has not studied it directly, but they have found that their predictions are not related to time of day. However, attention can fluctuate minute by minute and hour by hour, so it could be informative to capture data from an individual at multiple time points in a specific day. Another participant remarked that people who are depressed or lonely tend to pay attention to the negative, such as being hypervigilant to social threats. Rosenberg noted that sustained attention is not always a positive quality—it is important to pay attention, but not to the extent that it prevents response to other cues in the environment. Going forward, it will be important to characterize the brain signatures of different types of attention without assuming that "more is always better."

## ROLE OF MEDITATION IN IMPROVING BRAIN HEALTH AND RESILIENCE

Elizabeth Hoge discussed brain health and resilience in the context of research on meditation, a practice that is becoming increasingly popular and which is thought to confer health benefits. Her presentation was framed around how meditation training may improve brain health and resilience, with a focus on potential biological changes that may be detected as a result of meditation training.

### Effect of Meditation on Brain Structure

Hoge described cross-sectional research efforts to measure the effects of meditation using structural MRI to evaluate the density of brain matter in the cortex of meditators (Lazar et al., 2005). The study included 20 experienced meditators with an average of 9 years of daily meditation practice and 15 nonmeditating controls matched on age, sex, race, and education. The structural MRI showed several areas of significantly increased cortical thickness in the meditators compared to the controls.

Specifically, the brain areas of higher density in meditators were the insula and the prefrontal cortex. The insula is associated with interoception—or increased awareness of the body—which is in keeping with the aim of many meditation practices of paying attention to what is happening in the body. The insula is associated with the integration of sensory and emotional information as well as empathy and compassion; this area is also more active during compassion meditation (Lutz et al., 2008). The insula tends to be abnormal in people who have brain pathologies, Hoge added. For instance, the insula tends to be smaller in people with schizophrenia or bipolar disorder. The prefrontal cortex is associated with working memory, executive function, selective attention, and fluid intelligence. Plotting the age of the study participants revealed that control subjects had a standard decline in cortical thickness that would be expected with aging; however, the meditators did not show that decline. The research group postulated that meditation may help to slow normal aging through some type of protective effect or enhancement of resilience.

Another study looked at experienced yoga practitioners, meditators, and controls (Gard et al., 2014). The subjects' fluid intelligence was measured by Raven's Advanced Progressive Matrices. When the subjects' fluid intelligence was plotted against their ages, the typical decline of fluid intelligence with increased age was seen in the control subjects, with less decline among the meditators and experienced yoga practitioners. These studies suggest that there is a protective element to these practices, said Hoge. She noted that this is aligned with the ethos of the meditation tradition, which is designed to see reality more clearly and therefore help humans reach happiness and joy.

## Effect of Meditation on Resilience

Next, Hoge presented evidence related to the effect of meditation on resilience. The dictionary defines resilience as the ability to return to original shape after being stretched, pressed, bent, and so on, as well as recovering from and adjusting well to misfortune or change. In psychology, the concept of resilience refers to the ability of most people, when exposed even to extraordinary levels of stress and trauma, to maintain normal psychological and physical functioning and avoid serious mental illness (Russo et al., 2012).

### *Measuring Resilience in Humans*

Several strategies can be used to measure resilience in humans: (1) examining people who have experienced adversity, stress, or trauma and then function well later; (2) bringing people into the laboratory, stressing them, and then measuring their ability to cope; or (3) administering self-report questionnaires. The third strategy is the most commonly used to measure resilience in the available literature. Hoge carried out an informal analysis of the most recent 20 articles in PubMed on human psychological resilience. Only one-quarter of the subjects measured resilience in terms of mental or physical health outcomes after adversity; three-quarters measured resilience using pencil-and-paper self-report questionnaires. This is a concern, she said, because the latter strategy has never been validated against behavioral resilience as measured by the first or second strategies. Thus, it is not clear what this most common strategy is actually measuring.

These questionnaires, which typically are based on resilience scales constructed by psychometricians, are often used to evaluate the putative and vaguely defined construct of *resilience* related to the outcome of behavioral or pharmacological interventions. For example, one study concluded that treatment with tiagabine, fluoxetine, sertraline, and cognitive behavioral therapy improves resilience as measured by a self-administered questionnaire (Davidson et al., 2005). This underscores the problems related to measurement and reporting of resilience and the need to move the field toward validating these commonly used pencil-and-paper measures against some kind of behavioral measure.

### *Effect of Mindfulness Meditation on Resilience*

Hoge's laboratory carried out a study to assess the effect of mindfulness meditation practice on resilience. Beyond merely measuring resilience, the aim was to determine if the meditation practice actually improves a person's ability to cope in the face of adversity. Mindfulness meditation is a form of meditation with a focus on self-regulating one's attention—meaning, maintaining focus on the immediate experience of sensations, emotions, and thoughts in the present moment—and on adopting a particular orientation toward one's experiences in the present moment, which is characterized by curiosity, openness, and acceptance (Bishop et al., 2004).

Specifically, the researchers were interested in exploring the effect of mindfulness-based stress reduction in people with generalized anxiety disorder (Hoge et al., 2013a). See Box 4-2 for the *Diagnostic and Statistical Manual of Mental Disorders, Fifth Edition* (DSM-5) criteria for this disorder. The study design randomized about 90 participants either to a mindfulness-based stress reduction class or to an attention control group that received stress management education, which was an exact match for time, attention, and other variables in order to reduce expectancy bias and social effects in the meditation group. The outcome measures included (1) clinical anxiety symptoms; (2) acute stress measures during a laboratory stress task, including the self-reported State–Trait Anxiety Inventory (STAI) and endocrine measures; and (3) neuroimaging findings during an emotional face task. The researchers chose to measure resilience in terms of emotional reactivity to stress in a laboratory setting using the Trier Social Stress Test.[6] Participants completed the Trier Social

[6] The Trier Social Stress Test uses public speaking to induce stress in study participants by asking them to deliver an impromptu 8-minute speech in front of an audience of "evalu-

**BOX 4-2**
**DSM-5 Criteria for Generalized Anxiety Disorder**

- Frequent worry that is difficult to control
- And three of these:
  - Restlessness or feeling keyed up or on edge
  - Being easily fatigued
  - Difficulty concentrating or mind going blank
  - Irritability
  - Muscle tension
  - Sleep disturbance (difficulty falling asleep or staying asleep or restless, unsatisfying sleep)
- Functional impairment or distress
- Not attributable to other disorder or medical condition

SOURCE: American Psychiatric Association, 2013.

Stress Test twice, once prior to any intervention and 10 weeks later after the intervention.

Hoge reported that the meditation group had a significantly greater decrease in their STAI anxiety scores during their speech compared to the control group. Because they reported having less anxiety during the second test, it could mean that they are more resilient to stress after the mindfulness-based stress reduction class. Both before and after the intervention, participants also completed a questionnaire composed of self-statements during public speaking; they were asked the extent to which they agreed with different positive and negative statements about their speeches during the Trier test[7] (Hofmann and Dibartolo, 2000). After the intervention, people in the meditation group had a greater decrease in negative self-statements, although it was not statistically significant. However, there was a significant increase in the positive self-statements among the meditation group compared to the controls, despite the fact that the meditation training did not specifically teach participants to encourage themselves and did not contain any training in how to deal with the speech task. She surmised that this finding suggests that there

ators" wearing white lab coats. The test also includes a surprise arithmetic task that is assessed in real time by the evaluators.

[7] Example negative statements: "I'm a loser"; "A failure in this situation would be more proof of my incapacity." Example positive statements: "I can handle everything"; "This is an awkward situation but I can handle it."

is a potential component of resilience that might be described as treating oneself with more kindness or with more self-regard.

The researchers looked at changes in the levels of stress hormones in the two groups before and after the training intervention. They focused on the adrenocorticotropic hormone (ACTH) because it comes from the brain, unlike cortisol, and has a much shorter half-life that allows for greater temporal specificity. They assessed the two groups' differences in ACTH levels in response to the Trier test administered prior to and after the intervention. People in the meditation group had a statistically significant decreased overall ACTH response compared to the people in the control group, indicating that this group had decreases in stress hormones in addition to decreases in self-reported stress after mindfulness-based stress reduction training.

### Effect of Mindfulness Training on the Biology of the Brain

Hoge's research group has also looked at the longitudinal changes in the brains of people who have been taught how to meditate in order to assess which of those neural changes may underlie clinical benefits of mindfulness-based stress reduction in people with generalized anxiety disorder (Hölzel et al., 2013). The study was based on existing knowledge about generalized anxiety disorder (Maslowsky et al., 2010; Mennin et al., 2002, 2005). People with this disorder tend to have low emotion regulation ability, as manifested in more negative reactivity and poorer understanding of emotion. However, psychotherapy can improve emotion regulation ability, which is thought to result from the involvement of the prefrontal cortex when the amygdala is hyperreactive.

Study participants with generalized anxiety disorder were randomized to receive either mindfulness-based stress reduction or the control training. Before and after the intervention, participants completed an fMRI affect labeling task by making a determination about the emotion being presented in photographs with subjects displaying different facial expressions. The participants' fMRI responses to neutral facial expressions was of particular interest, because people with anxiety disorders tend to focus on and worry about the meaning of neutral or ambiguous information. The investigators carried out a functional connectivity analysis of the participants to measure the extent to which different brain regions coactivate, using the right amygdala as a seed.

Figure 4-3 illustrates how the changes that occurred as a result of the training were significantly different in the meditation group compared to the control group.

Panel B depicts the right superior frontal area, which is associated with social exclusion, social pain, and pain catastrophizing. Panel A

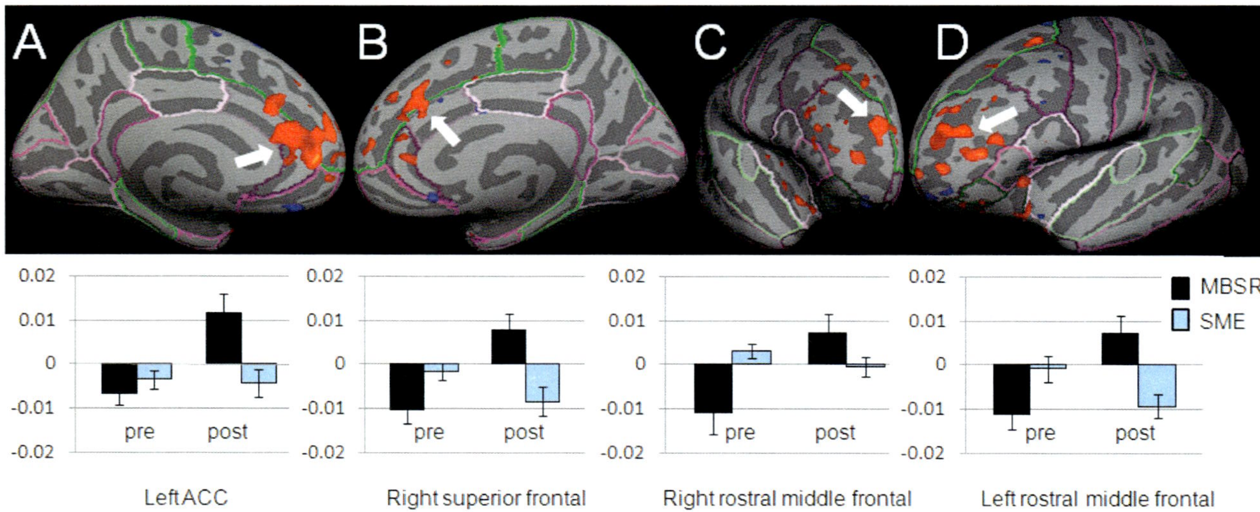


**FIGURE 4-3** Change in functional connectivity in patients with generalized anxiety disorder.
NOTE: ACC = anterior cingulate cortex; MBSR = mindfulness-based stress reduction; SME = stress management education.
SOURCES: As presented by Elizabeth Hoge at the workshop Brain Health Across the Life Span on September 24, 2019; adapted from Hölzel et al., 2013.

shows the significant changes in the anterior cingulate cortex, which forms part of the salience network with the insula; this subgenual part of the anterior cingulate cortex is associated with emotional regulation and affective tasks. Panels C and D show the prefrontal cortex areas. Panel C indicates that the same area of the cortex is associated with two different—but perhaps related—phenomena: it was involved when people with generalized anxiety disorders learned meditation, and was also found to be of greater thickness in experienced meditators. Next, investigators correlated the participants' Beck Anxiety Inventory scores after the intervention with their functional connectivity to evaluate the effect of these observed changes on clinical anxiety symptoms.

### Effect of Meditation on Longevity

Hoge concluded by describing her group's work using longevity as a measure for overall health by looking at telomere length in experienced meditators (Hoge et al., 2013b). Telomeres are caps at the ends of chromosomes that protect the tip of a chromosome from deterioration. They shorten with each replication and shorten predictably with age. According to cross-sectional data, telomere shortening appears to be accelerated in populations that experience increased psychological stress, such as mothers caring for a chronically ill child (Epel et al., 2004) or daughters of depressed mothers (Gotlib et al., 2015). The researchers predicted that longer telomeres would be observed in people who meditate if meditation is indeed protective, especially if they practice loving-kindness meditation. The study design was based on the presumption that being kind toward others can improve a person's overall health.

Other-focused activities such as community volunteering (Oman et al., 1999) and spousal caregiving (Brown et al., 2009) can sometimes improve health. Forgiveness of others is associated with greater longevity (Toussaint et al., 2012), and people with high hostility levels have a higher risk of mortality (Smith et al., 2004). The researchers recruited long-term meditators with experience in a type of meditation called loving-kindness meditation, or Metta, as well as controls matched on any factor that could affect telomeres. As expected, the loving-kindness meditators had longer telomeres than their age- and gender-matched controls. Overall, this difference was not significant. However, when broken down by gender, loving-kindness meditators who were women had significantly longer telomeres than their age-matched controls.

## Discussion

Colleen McClung, professor of psychiatry and clinical and translational science at the University of Pittsburgh, asked if study participants with anxiety ever report that mindfulness is counterproductively more stressful for them. Hoge said that in a clinical setting, meditation teachers specifically address this issue, which tends to help prevent catastrophizing types of thought cycles in the participants. However, some patients with posttraumatic stress disorder who experience flashbacks need to have exposure therapy first before learning how to meditate.

It has been suggested that it is the luxury of having quiet time to oneself that makes meditation and mindfulness beneficial for some people, McClung added. The data suggest that more is happening in meditation than time to oneself, said Hoge. In her study, people in the control group were also given audio tapes to listen to during their time to themselves that were unrelated to meditation. She suggested that there are active mechanisms specific to meditation that have to do with positive self-regard or being nonjudgmental, for instance. A participant asked Hoge to elaborate on dose response in the context of meditation (e.g., differences related to the length of experience meditating or the frequency of meditation). Hoge said that a significant dose–response relationship has not yet been established in the literature.

Akil commented about the use of the Trier Social Stress Test as described in Hoge's studies. Akil's group ran a study that looked at the effect of emotion on memory. Participants included people with depression, people with anxiety and depression, and healthy controls. They administered the Trier Social Stress Test and measured neuroendocrine markers, including ACTH, then did a follow-up study 1 or 2 weeks later to ask participants what they remembered about the experience. The participants with depression had better recall about their perceived failures in the arithmetic task, even though the group's actual error rate was no different—and in some cases even better—than the control group, who hardly remembered the test at all.

After this study, Akil stopped administering the Trier test in people with depression because of its traumatizing effect. She added that the ACTH response was not predictive in the group with depression, who tended to walk into the test with very high glucocorticoid levels because they were anticipating nervousness. Consequently, they tended to manifest a flat stress response instead of the solid response observed in controls. Harkening back to the distinction between good stress and bad stress, she noted that a solid stress response that starts and ends swiftly is preferable to a "floppy" response that never really ends, as is common among people with anxiety. In the context of defining resilience, she added, it is important to consider how long a negative reaction persists.

She suggested that memory of positive versus negative experiences could be used as one potential measure of resilience.

## PANEL DISCUSSION ON BEHAVIORAL AND BIOLOGICAL CONVERGENCE

Akil opened the discussion by asking panelists how they would define resilience based on their own research. Hoge replied that resilience relates to the capacity to cope with stress. A person experiencing bad stress may feel overwhelmed and lacking in the resources to cope, while a person experiencing good stress believes they have the resources to cope with it. Resilience could thus be defined by a person's belief in his or her ability to cope and succeed in the face of stress without negative mental or physical health outcomes. Within this paradigm, it could be useful to help people transform bad stress into good stress so they feel more confident and capable without being preoccupied by their past mistakes. Rosenberg suggested thinking about resilience as it changes over time, because it seems to involve dynamic processing to "bounce back" after a challenging situation.

The most difficult step in research on the brain and cognitive processes is to identify whether a given brain phenomenon is a risk factor or a response, said Damien Fair, associate professor of behavioral neuroscience, associate professor of psychiatry, and associate scientist at the Advanced Imaging Research Center at the Oregon Health & Science University. Differentiating between the two, while challenging, is critical for characterizing the brain's response to stress and how to manage it to improve long-term outcomes.

Gagan Wig, associate professor of behavioral and brain sciences at the Center for Vital Longevity at the University of Texas at Dallas, remarked that it might be useful to frame the discussion by considering a potential distinction between emotional and cognitive resilience. Cognitive resilience could be described as a system that is perturbed by some life event, but the system is still able to function on a longer time scale. In other words, cognitive resilience amounts to neurodegeneration that does not result in a major collapse of cognitive abilities, as opposed to organic damage of some kind.

It would be interesting to explore the extent to which different types of resilience are separable and how they feed into each other, said Akil. This could help inform strategies to help people with a low capacity for one type of resilience and a strong capacity for the other to use one to strengthen the other, possibly through cognitive therapy. When people's cognitive abilities decrease with age, for example, they may call on other neural circuitry to help with a declining function such as memory. She asked whether other types of capabilities could be called into action to compensate for or complement other types. Fair suggested that brain resilience is another distinction. The brain has the capacity to change as a function of various kinds of inputs; finding ways to measure that type of resilience would allow for better understanding of the capacity of the brain to be resilient in different contexts.

With regard to breaking out multiple types of resilience, Lis Nielsen, chief of the Individual Behavioral Processes Branch of the Division of Behavioral and Social Research at the National Institute on Aging, remarked that resilience is not limited to a particular part of the brain or physiology. It is likely that the brain has multiple capacities and systems that are related to resilience. She was concerned that striving for a single unifying definition of resilience—in the service of identifying specific measurable psychological capacities—could occlude the idea that resilience constitutes multiple capacities that interact with each other. Akil remarked that gene expression profiling over multiple brain regions in people with severe depression reveals a host of changes all throughout the brain—not just in one place. In those brains, the correlation of gene expression between regions has completely shifted, connections between reward circuits in the prefrontal cortex are altered, the balance of brain circuits has become tilted, and there is degradation of the support system at the biological level. When the symptoms of a brain disorder are this severe, it can be difficult to distinguish between affective, cognitive, attentional, and memory symptoms.

Akil suggested that understanding more about the sequence of events that lead to severe brain disorders could help to elucidate critical points of intervention. This knowledge could also shed light on integrative ways to help balance brain capacities that are undermined with brain capacities that are stronger. This underscores the idea that no single pattern of brain phenotypes or behavioral phenotypes can be used to achieve a healthy outcome or a healthy life, said Rosenberg (Holmes and Patrick, 2018). Instead, there are probably ways in which each person's phenotypes are more and less optimal, but they can operate together to produce good outcomes—there is a diversity of ways to achieve a healthy brain.

### Self-Report as a Measure of Resilience

Nielsen noted that although the scales that measure resilience are not necessarily well validated with real outcomes, self-report measures may be more suitable for assessing certain outcomes of resilient processing in response to an imposed stressor. For example, using experience sampling approaches to capture self-reported emotion over time—in parallel with measures that capture fluctuations in hormone levels or behavior—may offer insights about how people "bounce back" from a stressor or challenge. This is more informative than the scale-based self-reports that are widely used. Rosenberg commented that a component of resilience—how a person feels about their own abilities to handle a stressful situation—might only be measurable via self-report. Self-report scales are confounded by social desirability, noted Hoge, which can make a person's self-report inconsistent with how the person actually acted in a situation.

### Brain Imaging Signatures of Attention

Akil asked Rosenberg if the "healthy" style of attention has a particular brain imaging signature. She replied that there is no single signature for attention overall, nor is there a single ideal marker of the best kind of attention in every context. Rather, attention is composed of multiple different processes. Each person may have an attention vector, with a number of different overlapping networks—or perhaps even distinct networks—that predict different attentional processes (e.g., sustained attention, spatial orienting, alerting, executive control). Thus, each person has a different pattern of abilities and of functional networks related to those abilities. No single pattern is necessarily best in all contexts, so attention needs to be adjusted and deployed in a context-dependent way. For instance, the attentional demands of sitting in a lecture are very different than the attentional demands of navigating a dark forest at night. Being able to flexibly deploy attention is a skill in and of itself, Rosenberg added, so it is not always the case that there is one ideal marker of the best kind of attention in every context.

### Self-Awareness of Resilience and Other Brain Processes

Stephanie Cacioppo, director of the brain dynamics laboratory, assistant professor of psychiatry and behavioral neuroscience, and assistant professor at the Grossman Institute for Neuroscience at the University of Chicago Pritzker School of Medicine, asked other participants if people need to be aware that they are resilient in order to be resilient—meaning, have meta-awareness of their own resilience. In Cacioppo's brain dynamics studies, they have explored brain signatures of self-awareness. Cacioppo's team uses high-density electroencephalography (EEG) to measure how fast a person detects negative information or positive information. If the subject is lonely, within 200 milliseconds their brain will detect the difference between a threat and a positive event, but self-report questionnaires show that they are not aware that they have detected it. Hoge suggested that people who are resilient would generally be aware of it, and they would be able to self-report less stress in the face of a challenge or adversity. Fair said that people are not aware or cognizant of those types of dynamics in their own brains.

Akil remarked that brain measures could play an important role in gathering evidence of what is happening in the brain—beyond a person's awareness or consciousness—that could inform our understanding of our own health, vulnerability, and resilience toward achieving better well-being. She asked, "What are we missing, if we only look at behavior and not look at the brain?" Rosenberg noted that people are not always aware of their own attention lapses, but they can be detected with fMRI. The emerging field of real-time neurofeedback detects patterns in the brain related to certain processes and provides feedback to the person about that activity. Initial evidence suggests that this may be more effective than some behavioral interventions, she added (deBettencourt et al., 2015). The Western-style concept of brain function is very top down, noted Akil, but more Eastern philosophies, including meditation, have a more bottom-up way of looking at affective and cognitive control that is very autonomic, but also relates to immune function and peripheral input. She urged participants not to restrict their thinking to achieving resilience through conscious cognitive mechanisms.

Hoge replied that this is important to bear in mind, because people are not always able to articulate what they have experienced or why they experience life differently after doing meditation training. Brain imaging suggests that feelings are not being suppressed; instead, there was more connectivity between the prefrontal cortex and amygdala. Akil also highlighted the interaction between the cognitive and the affective—"Do we feel differently when we think differently, or do we think differently when we feel differently?" Rosenberg suggested that an interesting approach would be to try to predict individual differences in emotional processing or emotional resilience, to explore whether there are networks that predict those processes, and, if so, to look at the degree to which they overlap with networks involved in cognitive and attentional processes.

## Measuring Resilience

Akil asked the panelists to comment on executive function—or the ability to "shift gears"—in terms of resilience. It will be important, albeit challenging, to measure the brain's capacity for resilience, particularly in response to a given input or some genetic risk factor, said Fair. Rosenberg suggested a longitudinal approach: using a brain measure at baseline to predict an expected resilience outcome. Hoge was concerned that such an approach would not capture the "bouncing back" aspect of resilience, because it would measure a person's response in the face of a stressor, rather than the person's ability to recover.

## Gender Differences in Brain Disorders

Recent studies have shown that men and women with depression have almost opposite signatures in their brain, with different gene expression changes occurring in very different directions, said McClung. It also appears as if the inflammatory processes of depression mainly occur in men and not necessarily in women, suggesting that there may be sex-based differences in brain disorders to be explored further. Hoge noted that a very persistent finding in meditation treatment research is that it has a bigger effect in women, although it is not clear why. Akil said that an important research question is to better understand the sex or other types of individual differences in the effect of brain diseases, in resilience, in coping styles, and in different affective patterns, cognitive patterns, and attentional patterns. Ideally, the results would coalesce to reveal different "brain neurotypes" with respective features, characteristics, and functions. Certain neurotypes might make a person more responsive to meditation or to attention shifting in other ways, for example. A major challenge, however, will be to unpack the heterogeneity in a way that is positive and does not fall back on prescriptive labeling that could potentially be damaging. Better biological markers would be helpful in reframing research questions to help people improve their resilience and well-being, Hoge added.

# 5

# Measuring Brain Health

**Key Points Highlighted by Workshop Participants**

- Achieving the dream of precision neuroscience will require avoiding potholes by improving reproducibility, improving predictive modeling (particularly for the development of biomarkers), and better understanding intraindividual variability over time so it can be couched within the context of a person's life. (Russell Poldrack)
- Small sample sizes in neuroimaging studies undercut the ability to believe a significant number of the results coming out of the brain health literature; mandatory preregistration would contribute substantially to moving toward a neuroscience that is aimed at translating findings into more effective treatments. (Russell Poldrack)
- Purely behavioral or purely psychological measures can achieve the same standard of quality as a biological measure (Lis Nielsen), but measures and definitions should be arrived at through empiricism and evidence rather than through opinion. (Huda Akil)
- A person who is resilient could be defined as (1) having a variety of neurocognitive tools and networks that can be activated in the context of internal and external environmental

and psychological challenges, and (2) being able to adaptively activate these tools and networks to optimize function in response to environmental and psychological challenges. (Luke Stoeckel)

- Resilience could be framed as the ability to bring a wide range of cognitive tools to bear in challenging situations. In a sense, resilience is the opposite of test-retest reliability: people with more flexibility in their cognitive toolkit will look less like themselves from time point to time point. He suggested treating this variability and flexibility as a phenotype. (Russell Poldrack)
- Resilience can be defined as maintaining access to a sufficient range of cognitive tools and an adequate degree of neuroplasticity over time. The ability to "roll with the punches" and rebound from adversity, for example, partly depends on having more than one coping strategy available. However, this personalized definition does pose certain challenges for measuring brain health, because it would require individualized measurement of a person's cognition. (Huda Akil)

This chapter features a presentation on grand views and potholes on the road to precision neuroscience by Russell Poldrack, Albert Ray Lang Professor of Psychology at Stanford University. He discussed the methodological techniques and standards for reliability that are necessary for measuring brain health and resilience; he also described how quality metrics and criteria can improve measurement of brain health and resilience in future research.

## GRAND VIEWS AND POTHOLES ON THE ROAD TO PRECISION NEUROSCIENCE

Poldrack sketched an optimistic dream for the use of neuroscience around brain health as well as identifying challenges that may hinder achieving that vision. Achieving the dream of precision neuroscience will require avoiding potholes by improving reproducibility, improving predictive modeling (particularly for the development of biomarkers), and better understanding intraindividual variability over time so it can be couched within the context of a person's life. He opened by laying out the idea of precision medicine, defined as prevention and treatment strategies that take into account individual variability in genetics, environments, and lifestyles (Goossens et al., 2015). Precision medicine promises to provide targeted treatments that are more effective for everyone than one-size-fits-all treatments designed for the average patient. In recent years, substantial efforts have been devoted to developing this concept, including the 2015 Precision Medicine Initiative launched by the White House.[1] This wave is being driven in part by success stories emerging from precision cancer drugs that are markedly improving outcomes based on genetic targeting and treatment. For example, Gleevec is a precision cancer treatment developed for people with a particular genetic mutation that causes chronic myeloid leukemia. This drug can improve survival drastically—from 30 percent 5-year survival to almost 90 percent 5-year survival.[2] We are seeing this substantial improvement in outcomes in several other aspects of cancer and other diseases, as well.

Poldrack reflected on an optimistic dream of how a future precision neuroscience of brain health might process information from neuroscientific and other biological measurements to target the way that individuals are treated. A person who visits a physician with some kind of complaint related to cognitive or neurocognitive function would receive a range of tests that might involve imaging, genomics, gut microbiome analysis, or other new technologies. The test results would be analyzed by a complicated, indecipherable machine-learning system to generate specific recommendations about what the person can do to improve brain health—be it a medication, a particular diet, a certain type of exercise, or transcranial magnetic stimulation, for example. As a counterpoint to this optimistic vision, Poldrack cautioned that there are three "potholes" along the road to achieving the dream of precision neuroscience: (1) irreproducibility of results, (2) use of faulty predictive models, and (3) lack of understanding of intraindividual variability.

## The Reproducibility Crisis

Poldrack explained that a focus on reproducibility is emerging in other domains of individualized precision medicine, because the reproducibility crisis undercuts the degree to which the results in the current literature can be believed. The reproducibility crisis is a phenomenon described by John Ioannidis in his seminal 2005 paper on why most published research findings are false (Ioannidis, 2005). Ioannidis pointed out three features that drive higher or lower reproducibility in a particular

[1] See https://obamawhitehouse.archives.gov/precision-medicine (accessed November 18, 2019).

[2] See https://www.cancer.gov/research/progress/discovery/gleevec (accessed November 18, 2019).

area of study. The first is the size of studies: the larger the number of studies conducted in a field, the more likely their findings are to be true. The second factor is the number of tested relationships in a field, with the likelihood of findings being true decreasing as the number of tested relationships increases. The third factor relates to flexibility in designs, definitions, outcomes, and methods of analysis—greater flexibility decreases the likelihood that findings are true.

A study published by Drysdale et al. (2016) in *Nature* used resting-state functional magnetic resonance imaging (fMRI) to define connectivity biomarkers that define neurophysiological subtypes of depression. Using this technique to cluster participants revealed that individuals with depression seem to have impairments in connectivity in different brain systems; the groups also differed substantially in their response to transcranial stimulation treatment. Although a replication of the full study has not yet been attempted, another group tried and failed to replicate the particular connectivity feature showed in the Drysdale study (Dinga et al., 2019). This reflects broader concerns about imaging studies: (1) a lack of understanding about what replicates and (2) the inability to replicate results.

### *Insufficient Scanning Time*

Estimating connectivity reliably requires substantial scan time, but the brain imaging studies currently being carried out are collecting far too little information about each individual. Poldrack estimated that achieving reliable measurements of connectivity requires something in the range of 30–100 minutes of resting-state data from a subject, depending on the degree of reliability desired, but most studies collect less than 10 minutes of resting-state data (Laumann et al., 2015). For instance, the Drysdale study collected an average range of 4.5–10 minutes of data from each subject. This underlines the need to further investigate how the amount of data studies collect from each individual relates to the reliability of the results.

At a group level, findings across brain imaging literature are not sufficiently reliable, said Poldrack. A number of meta-analyses looked at around 100 neuroimaging studies of depression and reported that there are significant differences in brain activity between people diagnosed with depression and healthy individuals (Müller et al., 2017). However, a research group with great expertise in neuroimaging meta-analysis performed a conceptual replication of the previous work. Across those same 100 studies, the group found no convergent differences in brain activity between healthy and depressed individuals, which was directly at odds with the findings of the previous meta-analyses (Müller et al., 2017).

*Underpowered Studies with Insufficient Sample Sizes*

The issues highlighted by Ioannidis are at the forefront of concerns about neuroimaging, said Poldrack. A large proportion of neuroscience research is badly underpowered across both human structural neuroimaging studies and animal studies, undermining the reliability of neuroscience research (Button et al., 2013). If a study has less than 10 percent power, it means that even if there is an effect, it will only be found 10 percent of the time. Although controlling for type-1 error can help control the false-positive rate, it does not mean that positive findings will necessarily be true.

The primary focus of research should not be the number of positive findings but how many of those positive findings are actually true. Positive predictive value is the probability that a positive result is true (Button et al., 2013). Statistical power substantially affects the ability to believe positive results that are published in the literature, Poldrack emphasized. In addition to being more likely to generate false results, underpowered studies are also more likely to produce results in which the effect sizes are overestimated. The overestimation of effect sizes for significant results is known as the Winner's Curse.

To illustrate the concept of positive predictive value, Poldrack described the following hypothetical scenario:

> Imagine you are going to do 100 studies, but your detector is broken so you only have random noise. If you controlled the false-positive rate at 5 percent, then on average, five of those 100 studies will come out with significant results. But the positive predictive value—the likelihood of the proportion of those positive results that are true—is zero, because the detector is broken. If the detector is fixed, then it will begin to capture true signals, then the positive predictive value will increase.

Poldrack plotted the sample sizes from the studies from the Müller et al. (2017) depression imaging meta-analysis as a function of year of publication. Current practice for reproducible research holds that 20 observations is a fundamental baseline for a study to be powerful enough to detect most effects (Simmons et al., 2011). Unless there is a compelling cost-of-data-collection justification, it does not make sense to collect fewer than 20 observations. In general, published data with a sample size of 20 tends to reflect a more flexible sample size determination based on interim data analysis and other types of problematic analyses. A majority of studies in the meta-analysis had grossly insufficient *N*. In other words, researchers invited more than 600 people with depression to volunteer for fMRI studies that were almost certain to generate either null or false results because of insufficient power.

This issue abounds in the brain health literature, said Poldrack. He carried out an informal search on PubMed for the terms *brain health* and *fMRI*, yielding 22 studies published in 2011 or later. Based on the published sample sizes for each group in each study, 22 percent of the groups included fewer than 20 subjects. This undercuts the ability to believe a significant number of the results coming out of the brain health literature, he cautioned. Poldrack suggested that mandatory preregistration would contribute substantially to moving toward a neuroscience that is aimed at translating findings into more effective treatments (see Box 5-1).

*Methodological Pluralism*

Methodological flexibility is a major challenge in the field of neuroimaging, because researchers have a large degree of flexibility in how they analyze neuroimaging data. One study analyzed a single event-related fMRI experiment using almost 7,000 different unique analysis procedures, in order to highlight the amount of variability seen across neuroimaging research (Carp, 2012). Poldrack's group is assessing the effects of this type of methodological pluralism in the Neuroimaging Analysis Replication and Prediction Study. They collected a dataset at Tel Aviv University on a

**BOX 5-1**
**Mandatory Preregistration**

Mandatory preregistration could help to propel neuroscience toward findings that can be translated into more effective treatments. This involves investigators preregistering their study plans—including sample size, inclusion or exclusion, analysis plan, and primary outcomes—prior to carrying out the study. This does not preclude exploratory analysis of data, but it does prevent those exploratory analyses from being presented as hypothesis driven (also called HARKing) and open to criticism. This practice helps to prevent unfounded claims of positive effects, as demonstrated in other areas of research. In 2000, the National Heart, Lung, and Blood Institute instituted a requirement that clinical trials for relevant drug or dietary supplement interventions must preregister the outcomes for which they will be looking. Prior to this policy, clinical trials largely claimed positive effects, with virtually no claims of harmful effect and relatively few claims of null effect. During those years, the flexibility built into the process allowed researchers to claim positive findings that were probably false in many cases. In the years since the policy was instituted, almost every study reports a null effect, with very few showing a beneficial effect and one trial even showing a harmful effect (Kaplan and Irvin, 2015).

SOURCE: As presented by Russell Poldrack at the workshop Brain Health Across the Life Span on September 24, 2019.

decision-making task and distributed the datasets to 82 different research groups, 70 of which returned their decisions on a set of given hypotheses[3] using their standard analysis methods, as well as providing thresholded and unthresholded maps. Economists helped to perform prediction markets to assess the researchers' abilities to predict outcomes. The findings of the study are still being prepared, but they have found that analytic variability leads to inconsistent results (Botvinik-Nezer et al., 2019). Even using exactly the same data in the reasonably well powered study, the variability across different groups in how the data are analyzed is substantial enough to drive a high degree of variability in the decisions that they make about particular hypotheses.

### Faulty Predictive Models

Poldrack turned to the pothole of faulty predictive models. Predictive models are essential to precision science, but faulty predictive models are another pothole on the roadway to precision neuroscience. A focus on developing biomarkers has been a rising trend in the neuroimaging literature over the past decade, yet many researchers tend to misrepresent the concept in a way that oversells it. A claim in favor of a biomarker is generally based on some claim about prediction. In the literature, people often make claims about prediction using an observed correlation or regression effect in a dataset. He deemed this move fundamentally problematic because the observed correlation within a dataset typically—in fact, almost always—overestimates the degree that a prediction can be made in a new dataset, because the data are being reused both to fit the model and to assess how well the model fits.

An observed correlation does not equate to predictive accuracy (Copas, 1983). This issue is known as *shrinkage* in statistics and as *overfitting* in machine learning. In machine learning, out-of-sample predictive accuracy is generally quantified using cross-validation with a different dataset. This process of cross-validation involves iteratively training a model on a subset of the data (the training data) and then testing the accuracy of the model's predictions on the remaining data (the validation data). Poldrack's group looked at the recent literature on fMRI, finding that about half of the publications claim putative "prediction," yet they are actually just demonstrating an in-sample correlation/regression effect within a single sample (Poldrack et al., 2019). The problem is that in-sample prediction inflates predictive accuracy. With increasing model complexity, in-sample prediction can be significant even with no true signal. However, using cross-validation or new data reveals that what looks

[3] For example, "Is there activation in area X for contrast Y in this study?"

like significant classification accuracy is actually the result of overfitting to the training data.

Small samples also inflate predictive accuracy estimates (Varoquaux, 2018). The decline of effect size over time and with respect to sample size is particularly problematic in the use of machine-learning tools (Varoquaux, 2018). In brain imaging, early studies with small sample sizes tended to claim very high predictive accuracy (even up to 100 percent) of psychiatric diagnoses based on imaging data. In almost every case, direct evidence shows that this was the result of using small samples (Varoquaux, 2018). Poldrack's group looked at sample sizes from publications claiming to show prediction based on fMRI, but more than half of the studies have sample sizes of less than 50 and 18 percent have sample sizes smaller than 20.[4] "Doing machine learning with sample sizes smaller than 20 is almost guaranteed to give you nonsense," he warned.

As the field of neuroscience moves toward greater appreciation of the problematic issues related to developing predictive models and how it may be contributing to the development of invalid biomarkers, it may be instructive to look to other fields to see their requirements for generating biomarkers. Biomarkers for cancer or other diseases are generally validated with very large samples of tens of thousands of samples. Damien Fair asked if studies with small sample sizes should be measuring cross-validation within the sample, or whether the same result is generated even with a small sample size for training and a completely independent dataset for testing. Poldrack replied that the results will be much more variable with a small sample size, but training on a small sample size and then testing on an independent small sample will help to modulate the variability and avoid overfitting.

### Poor Understanding of Intraindividual Variability Over Time

Poldrack turned to his third pothole on the road to precision neuroscience, which is poor understanding of intraindividual variability over time. An increasing body of knowledge is providing insight into how brain function changes over time on both ends of the spectrum from milliseconds to decades (Sowell et al., 2004). However, there is still a dearth of knowledge in the middle of the spectrum, with respect to how brain function changes across days, weeks, or months. It has become clear that understanding brain disorders requires understanding individual variability in brain function. A person with schizophrenia or bipolar disorder,

[4] Poldrack, R. Workshop presentation—Grand Views and Potholes on the Road to Precision Neuroscience. Available at http://www.nationalacademies.org/hmd/Activities/Aging/BrainHealthAcrossTheLifeSpanWorkshop/2019-JUN-26.aspx (accessed March 12, 2020).

for example, will tend to have significant fluctuations between high and low functional levels across daily life (Bopp et al., 2010). Over the course of a few weeks, an individual can go from completely disabled to reasonably functional (Kupper and Hoffmann, 2000). Labeling somebody as having a particular disorder glosses over the large degree of variability from day to day and week to week in how that disorder is being expressed.

Nearly all of human neuroscience assumes that the functional organization of the brain is stable outside of plasticity, development, and aging. But until very recently, this assumption has not been tested empirically. Understanding the variability and dynamics of human brain function at multiple time scales is critical for the development of precision neuroscience and neuroscientific interventions, he said. In 2013, Poldrack engaged in a study called the My Connectome project by collecting as much data about himself as possible, including imaging data from more than 100 scans (resting fMRI, task fMRI, diffusion MRI, and structural MRI), behavioral data (mood, lifestyle, and sleep), and other biological measurements (Laumann et al., 2015; Poldrack et al., 2015). They found that the pattern of variability between individuals is fundamentally different than the pattern of variability within individuals. They found high variability in Poldrack's primary sensory motor networks across sessions. Imaging studies across 120 individuals did reveal some variability in somatomotor and visual networks, but that was dwarfed by variability in default, frontoparietal, and dorsal attention networks.

This highlights the need to study individual variability in more depth, in order to identify factors that may drive variance in resting-state connectivity within an individual. The My Connectome project revealed that intake of caffeine and food affects large-scale network structure, for example (Poldrack et al., 2015). Figure 5-1 shows that on days in which he fasted and did not drink caffeine in the morning before the scan, his somatomotor network and the secondary visual network were highly connected; on mornings in which he consumed food and caffeine before the scan, those networks were essentially disconnected. He emphasized that this is not an overall degradation in connectivity—it is a real change in the structure of connectivity. This has serious implications regarding the effect of these types of factors on neuroimaging.

### *Longer-Scale Dynamics Within Individuals*

Evidence suggests that there are also longer-scale dynamics within individuals. An analysis of the data across the entire My Connectome session looked for patterns of connectivity recurring over time, and found two "temporal metastates" that were present throughout (Shine et al., 2016). Both seemed to be related to his being attentive, concentrating,

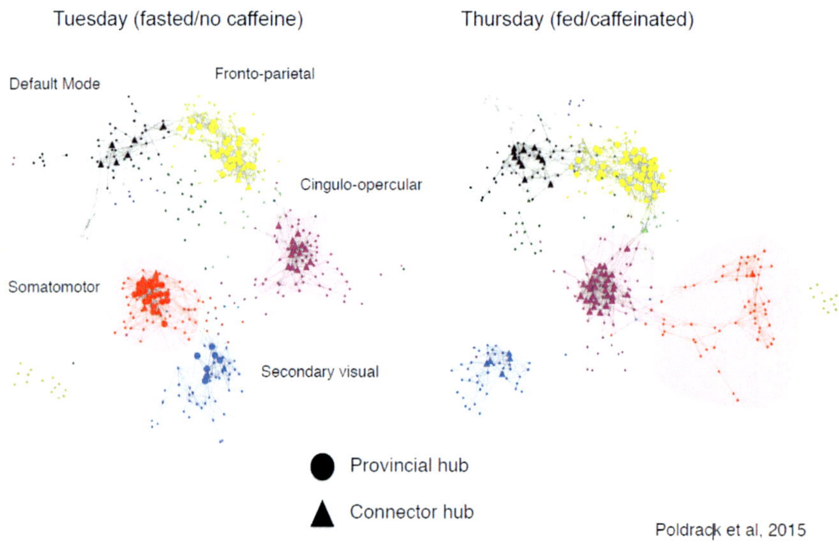


**FIGURE 5-1** Caffeine and food consumption affects large-scale network structure.
SOURCES: As presented by Russell Poldrack at the workshop Brain Health Across the Life Span on September 24, 2019; Poldrack et al., 2015.

or lively versus his being drowsy, sleepy, sluggish, or tired. These meta-states were not significantly correlated with caffeine or food intake. When he was drowsy or sluggish, there was much greater integration of the visual and somatomotor networks, while the other networks became slightly more concentrated on the days when he was fed and caffeinated. Despite the wealth of potential knowledge to be mined from these types of individual scanning studies, very little of this work has been done—the number of dense longitudinally scanned individuals remains at approximately less than 20. Denser data collection from individuals will need to increase in order to better understand variability at multiple scales with sufficient power. He suggested that the field of imaging should draw from the literature on aging about characterizing the dynamics of behavioral processes at multiple scales over time (Ram, 2015). Different forms of intraindividual variability are situated within the context of much longer scale intraindividual change, as well as interindividual variability.

## Discussion

Damien Fair, associate professor of behavioral neuroscience, associate professor of psychiatry, and associate scientist at the Advanced Imaging Research Center at the Oregon Health & Science University, asked about behavioral measurements assessing outcomes such as cognitive ability or clinical status. Poldrack replied that his group has recently published papers, including one on the nature and quality of behavioral measures used in the domain of self-regulation and self-control. He noted that measures used in experimental psychology are not typically focused on reliability to the same extent as survey measures, which are designed to be reliable. That study found that, as expected, survey measures had good reliability. On average, the behavioral measures had bad reliability, particularly those that were designed to measure contrasts in task performance across different conditions.

Generally, tasks used in cognitive psychology to isolate particular cognitive components are not useful as measures of individual differences. These types of measures, such as the Stroop task, can be useful and have a robust effect, but the effect is not robust at the level of test reliability; therefore, they are not reliable enough to provide any validity as an individual difference measure. Huda Akil, codirector and research professor of the Molecular and Behavioral Neuroscience Institute and Quarton Professor of Neurosciences at the University of Michigan, added that just because a measure is useful as a group measure, it is not necessarily good as an individual measure; this distinction is an important one that should be more prominently taught to researchers.

Akil remarked that the field of brain science has generated a large body of real and actionable knowledge, but it would be helpful to know where the failures lie; for example, as to whether the nature of the measurements, the level of analysis, the use of human versus animal models, and so on. Poldrack replied that for imaging purposes, certain findings about the organization of the brain are replicable and reliable. He drew a line, however, between group mean activation and correlation of individual differences and group differences. The real failures of reproducibility are being seen in differences between diagnostic and control groups, as well as in correlations across the individuals—simply because the sample sizes are far too small.

Part of the issue is measurement, but another issue is that insufficient data are being collected at the individual level. "We should not expect DSM-5 diagnoses to really cleanly carve the brain at its joints, because we know that they are not biologically coherent phenotypes," he said. Overlaid on these issues are the problems of analytic variability—because different methods of analyzing data will naturally lead to different results—and of publication bias, because journals are not willing to publish null results. This makes it tempting for researchers to perform many different analyses until one of them generates a non-null result. These issues are compounded in the context of underpowered studies on individual differences or group differences.

Gagan Wig, associate professor of behavioral and brain sciences at the Center for Vital Longevity at the University of Texas at Dallas, commented that identification of changes in measures of brain and behavior, or even assessment of reliability of measures of brain and behavior, could be confounded by differences in practice effects (unanticipated learning of the testing procedures), although he noted that this learning itself could also potentially provide an informative additional signal about individual variability. Poldrack replied that test-retest reliability could be useful if looking for a stable measure of an individual, but not if the intent is to be sensitive to change. The main idea is that the psychometric features of the task being used need to be appropriate for the construct that the study is attempting to measure. When building measures that are intended to be sensitive to learning, for example, it is important to ensure that the measures are reliably sensitive to learning—not necessarily in the test-retest sense, but perhaps in some other sense.

## PANEL DISCUSSION ON THE WAY FORWARD IN MEASUREMENT AND RESEARCH

Akil asked the panelists to reflect on key issues in measuring brain health. With the caveat that much more work is needed to define brain health as a construct that can be measured at all, Poldrack noted that the field has integrated the concept of big data in a very limited way—that is, collecting a small amount of data from a relatively large number of people. Ultimately, the ability to carry out large-scale analyses is limited by the quality of those individual measurements. More sensitivity is needed in the degree to which a stable phenotype is being measured at the individual level, even if it is just stable within a day. The field should also be looking across phenotypes, he said, by collecting many different measurements from the same individuals. Monica Rosenberg, assistant professor in the Department of Psychology at the University of Chicago, emphasized the importance of sharing and integrating data and models (including feature weights and prediction algorithms) to allow for external validation and help move the field toward the identification of real biomarkers.

### Research Domain Criteria Project

Elizabeth Hoge, director of the anxiety disorders research program at the Georgetown University Medical Center, noted that the Research Domain Criteria (RDoC)[5] project is an alternative framework for mental

[5] See https://www.nimh.nih.gov/research/research-funded-by-nimh/rdoc/index.shtml (accessed November 18, 2019).

illness than the *Diagnostic and Statistical Manual of Mental Disorders, 5th Edition* (DSM-5). It focuses more on the need to study and measure dimensions such as cognitive function and affective valence, for example, instead of focusing on measuring disease. The aim is that RDoC would yield more connections to biology and facilitate more translation between animal and human models. Fair said that RDoC is helpful in moving away from the discrete DSM categories, but it has its own limitations that will need to be addressed.

Akil expressed concern that like the DSM, the RDoC project was also developed by committee and is not biologically based, so one orthodoxy is essentially being replaced with another. The advantage of RDoC is that it encourages people to think in terms of function rather than disease; moving away from the disease-based approach will require considering dimensionality of different phenotypes. However, the RDoC project would benefit from being more biologically informed and appropriately validated. The reliability of measures will need to be established in order for biology to become the framework to inform treatment and prevention in the field of brain health, in keeping with the shift toward precision medicine.

Colleen McClung, professor of psychiatry and clinical and translational science at the University of Pittsburgh, remarked that the animal research community is struggling somewhat with the advent of RDoC. After much effort building animal models with various characteristics and brain–body features of psychiatric diseases, researchers are now being asked to study each characteristic in isolation. RDoC has been helpful in encouraging cognitive neuroscience to adopt a dimensional perspective, said Rosenberg. Symptoms exist on a continuum, so the dimensional approach of concrete predictive modeling of continuous measures of behavior or symptoms—or data-driven subtyping—can capture symptom variability and complement binary or categorical classifications. For example, predicting attention-deficit hyperactivity disorder (ADHD) symptoms yields significant prediction of symptoms even in people without ADHD diagnoses, reflecting the broader variability in attention function among healthy people.

Lis Nielsen, chief of the Individual Behavioral Processes Branch of the Division of Behavioral and Social Research at the National Institute on Aging, said that measures in psychological domains do not necessarily need to be derived from biology. They can be based on functional or behavioral categories; mental health and subjective states, for instance, can be assessed by self-report or performance-based tasks. Purely behavioral or purely psychological measures can achieve the same standard of quality as a biological measure. Akil clarified that she is calling for a system that is empirically evidence based, rather than committee based.

RDoC also harks back to the issue of trait versus state, said Akil. She believes that coping and affective disorders contain nested concepts that could be disentangled biologically, genetically, and environmentally. With a broad lens, the tendencies that we might call "temperament" are changeable, but fairly stable phenotypes. However, variability in features such as coping style or willingness to explore are adaptive for a species in an intermediate context—such as responding to stress during adolescence—or in moment-to-moment responses. These time-nested ways of thinking, including behaviorally and biologically, could be helpful in thinking about measurement. Poldrack said that the Midnight Scan Club data have shown that in general, connectivity patterns are quite stable within an individual. Rosenberg added that stable patterns have been observed consistently across several datasets that used high-frequency sampling of a small number of individuals, which bodes well for capturing models that predict trait-like behaviors.

McClung said that chronotypes are relatively stable after adolescence and before the age of 65 years or so. In fact, certain polymorphisms in circadian genes have been associated with traits of being a morning person or a nighttime person. Akil suggested that in the context of defining and measuring brain health, these are all examples of elements of the general framework or signature for how an individual is functioning; changes occur when things are either declining or improving.

## Defining Resilience

Luke Stoeckel, National Institutes of Health, proposed a two-part working definition of resilience in the context of brain health. A person who is resilient could be defined as (1) having a variety of neurocognitive tools and networks that can be activated in the context of internal and external environmental and psychological challenges, and (2) being able to adaptively activate these tools and networks to optimize function in response to environmental and psychological challenges. Poldrack suggested that resilience could be framed as the ability to bring a wide range of cognitive tools to bear in challenging situations. In a sense, resilience is the opposite of test-retest reliability: people with more flexibility in their cognitive toolkit will look less like themselves from time point to time point. He suggested treating this variability and flexibility as a phenotype. Akil sketched her own definition of resilience. Neuroplasticity is a finite resource, but there may be ways to increase or maintain reserves of neuroplasticity. Similarly, maintaining intellectual, emotional, and physical flexibility is a component of being resilient that speaks directly to having more affective or cognitive resources to draw upon.

In early life, the brain has a large degree of flexibility and many available options and tools, so the natural pruning that occurs is necessary. However, this pruning should not be excessive to the point of eliminating too many of those options and coping tools, which would preclude the ability to respond effectively to adversity. In this context, resilience can be defined as maintaining access to a sufficient range of cognitive tools and an adequate degree of neuroplasticity over time. The ability to "roll with the punches" and rebound from adversity, for example, partly depends on having more than one coping strategy available. However, this personalized definition does pose certain challenges for measuring brain health, because it would require individualized measurement of a person's cognition.

# 6

# Brain Health in the Social Context

**Key Points Highlighted by Workshop Participants**

- It has been posited that there are three different types of connections in an individual: intimate connections, relational connections, and collective connections. Further study is warranted to understand the relationships between those connections (or lack thereof) and loneliness. (Stephanie Cacioppo)
- Research on brain health cannot be conducted using convenience samples, which proliferates in research on older adult brain health. Selection bias is prevalent in studies that use clinic-based or convenience samples, in which participants are recruited from clinics that specialize in memory disorders. (Jennifer Manly)
- Brain health disparities research must measure life-course individual or contextual factors, such as social determinants of health or the social exposome, sufficiently well to determine the relative contributions of bio-psycho-behavioral-social factors to disease or interactions. Experts in quantifying brain health have not traditionally focused on social determinants of health across the life course. As a result, measurements of social determinants are often lacking even in studies that have exquisite measurements of brain health

outcomes. Variables related to the social determinants of health—including childhood exposures and administrative policies in educational systems—are crucial for understanding trajectories of brain health. Understanding the neuropathological mechanisms underlying brain health disparities will require studying people earlier in life. (Jennifer Manly)

- The research infrastructure could be strengthened by adding retrospective measures of social exposome variables to studies that focused on older age or by designing earlier life-course studies to incorporate those types of measures. Therefore, those measures will be valuable for long-term studies of aging and brain health. (Lis Nielsen)
- It is a future research challenge to develop harmonized measures, both of risk factors and of brain health outcomes; these are critical for combining cohorts, synthesizing research, and accelerating knowledge. (Jennifer Manly)
- Brain health can be thought about as (1) a person's accumulative reserve, which sets the intercept or starting point, and (2) the degree to which a person is affected by adversities, such as stress or the onset of illness. These adversities are likely to be related and difficult to tease apart unless they are measured from an early stage—from birth or even in utero. (Deanna Barch)

This chapter summarizes the workshop session on brain health in the social context, particularly with respect to both emotions and social disparities. Presenters and panelists looked at how an individual's social context affects his or her brain health and resilience, how various social factors are important for understanding and predicting brain health, and how those factors are measured and validated. Stephanie Cacioppo, assistant professor of psychiatry and behavioral neuroscience and assistant professor at the Grossman Institute for Neuroscience at the University of Chicago, provided an overview of how the brain forms, maintains, and restores healthy relationships. Gregory Samanez-Larkin, assistant professor of psychology and neuroscience at Duke University, examined motivation, cognition, and decision making in everyday life. Life-course causes of later-life inequalities in brain health were explored by Jennifer Manly, professor of neuropsychology at Columbia University.

## FROM ME TO WE: HOW THE BRAIN FORMS, MAINTAINS, AND RESTORES HEALTHY RELATIONSHIPS

Cacioppo described the improvement of brain health and social resilience as among the most important challenges facing contemporary science. When a 1978 report by the U.S. President's Commission on Mental Health emphasized the importance of easing suffering from emotional distress syndromes such as loneliness, few anticipated that this issue would persist more than 40 years later. The issue is gaining an increasing amount of attention, with the number of scientific papers published per year on loneliness increasing by roughly tenfold (Cacioppo and Cacioppo, 2018a). Cacioppo described what the former Surgeon General of the United States, Vivek Murthy, described as the loneliness epidemic.

People are living longer than ever before, with the rise of the Internet transforming how people work, play, search, shop, study, communicate, and relate to one another. People are increasingly connected digitally, but social media do not necessarily protect them from loneliness or perceived social isolation—it depends on how they are used. These platforms may reduce loneliness in people who use them to connect, learn, or stay in touch with loved ones, but in people who use social media to the extent that they have only online connections with others, feelings of loneliness can increase (Cacioppo et al., 2015b). The prevalence of loneliness appears to be rising, from an estimated 11–17 percent of adults in the 1970s to more than 40 percent of adults middle-aged and older in recent years (Edmondson, 2010; Peplau et al., 1979; Perissinotto et al., 2012).

### Defining and Measuring Loneliness

Loneliness is often discussed in conjunction with social resilience in publications. Social resilience is inherently a multilevel construct—revealed by capacities of individuals and also groups—to foster, engage in, and sustain positive social relationships and to endure and recover from social stressors and social isolation (Cacioppo et al., 2011). The premise underlying this work on loneliness and social resilience is that the brain is the main "social organ." It is a key organ for forming, monitoring, and maintaining healthy connections with others as well as for regulating physiological processes relevant to morbidity and mortality. The brain helps organize a person's social structures and social behaviors; it also regulates the social processes that determine health and longevity (Cacioppo and Cacioppo, 2018a).

People often think about humans as being unique compared to other species and think of themselves as unique and independent relative to those around them. Although individuals may appear to be distinct and independent, with no forces binding them together, people in fact have more similarities than differences. Humans are a social species that is wired to form social connections and maintain those connections across the life span (Cacioppo and Cacioppo, 2012). The brain is primarily responsible for forming, monitoring, and maintaining those salutary connections with others. To illustrate the difference between objective and subjective isolation, Cacioppo used the example of how the same objective social interaction or relationship (e.g., with a sibling or a spouse) can be perceived either as caring and protective or as threatening and isolating. A person can feel "lonely in a crowd" when public speaking, for instance, while a person can feel extremely connected while completely alone just by thinking about loved ones. Thus, loneliness can be defined as perceived social isolation: a discrepancy between current and expected social relationships with a significant other.

Several different scales can be used to measure loneliness, but three main items have been evaluated as consistently reliable measures (Cacioppo and Cacioppo, 2018a).

1. How often do you feel that you lack companionship?
2. How often do you feel left out?
3. How often do you feel isolated from others?

## Effect of Loneliness on Physical and Mental Health

As the prevalence of loneliness rises, more evidence is accruing that loneliness is a major risk factor for poor physical and mental health outcomes (Cacioppo and Cacioppo, 2018a). For instance, the odds ratio for dying earlier from loneliness has been shown to be much higher (45 percent) than from excessive drinking (30 percent), obesity (20 percent), or air pollution (5 percent) (Holt-Lunstad et al., 2010). Studies in animals or humans demonstrate the effect of loneliness or lack of social connection on both physical and mental health, including the activation of the stress response, increases in inflammatory mechanisms, and increases in cell deaths in specific brain areas. A quantitative meta-analysis of functional imaging studies of social rejection found that when people feel rejected, a specific set of brain areas is activated, although this can be modulated as a function of whether the person is rejected by a stranger or a significant other. All the activated brain areas were in the specific networks involved in emotions and in expectations by relation (Cacioppo et al., 2013). When a person feels lonely, a different set of brain areas activates or deactivates in the social brain networks instead: areas that are important for empathy, compassion, perspective taking, and being in synchrony with others (Cacioppo et al., 2014).

Evidence from different types of social species may cast light on the social dimension of the human brain. For instance, the locust shifts from solitary to social within a year; it has a brain that is about 30 percent larger when it is social than when it is nonsocial (Burrows et al., 2011; Ott and Rogers, 2010; Rogers and Ott, 2015). Studies using functional magnetic resonance imaging (fMRI) of people with different social network sizes have also revealed differences in sizes in various parts of the social brain (Cacioppo et al., 2014). Cacioppo emphasized that it is not the entire brain that increases in size, only the brain areas needed for social connections. When a locust is social, it only needs to communicate with olfactory senses or with touch, so the brain areas involved in motor sensory integration are bigger or more active. But when the locust is solitary, the visual cortex has greater activation because increased visual attention is needed to detect threats at a distance. Similarly, in humans, the visual cortex is also more activated in lonely individuals (Cacioppo et al., 2014). Cacioppo surmised that these individuals may have a hypervigilance to social threat or potential danger, and thus a hyperactivation in areas of the brain that are important for perspective taking, empathizing, or connecting with others.

### An Evolutionary Theory of Loneliness

It has long been understood that brain health and survival depend on our collective abilities, not our individual might, said Cacioppo. Decades of research in social psychology shows that happy marriages have myriad beneficial effects on health through behavioral, cardiovascular, neuroendocrine, immune system, and cognitive pathways. People who are married have fewer physical problems, a better survival rate for some illnesses, and a lower mortality rate (Cacioppo, 2018; Goodwin et al., 1987; Lillard et al., 1995; Murphy et al., 1997; Waite and Lehrer, 2003). Throughout history, humans have survived and prospered by bonding together in couples, families, and tribes—to provide companionship, mutual protection, and aid. However, marital status is not the main factor associated with better health; rather, it is the quality of the relationship with a significant other that is crucial (Cacioppo, 2018).

Working toward a consistent definition of "significant other" is challenging, but it could be informed by studies of different species. For instance, adult female baboons (>5 years of age) who form stronger and more stable social bonds with other females live significantly longer than females who form weaker and less stable relationships (Silk et al., 2010). Another study tested two species, monogamous titi monkeys and nonmonogamous squirrel monkeys (Mendoza and Mason, 1986). When researchers removed one of the significant monkeys from a group of polygamous monkeys, they observed no increase in cortisol in the remaining monkeys, presumably because the group could find another partner. When the researchers removed the offspring, however, they observed a large increase in plasma cortisol after 1 hour of separation. The opposite was found in the monogamous titi monkeys. When researchers removed a monkey from a monogamous pair, they saw a huge stress response after 1 hour, but not when they removed the offspring. This suggests that within the titi monkey's social hierarchy, the partner is more significant than the offspring.

Cacioppo suggested that evolutionary heritage has shaped the human brain and biology to be inclined toward certain ways of feeling, thinking, and acting toward significant others. For instance, a variety of biological mechanisms have evolved that capitalize on aversive signals to motivate behaviors that increase the chances of short-term survival. Within this framework of evolutionary theory, loneliness is like a biological signal in that the aversiveness of loneliness serves as a biological warning signal analogous to hunger, thirst, and pain. It motivates attention and the repair or replacement of deficiencies in salutary relationships. In other words, it signals that something is wrong with a person's "social body," so the person needs to reconnect with others in order to survive (Cacioppo and Cacioppo, 2014, 2018b; Cacioppo and Patrick, 2008; Cacioppo et al., 2000, 2006).

## Pathways of Loneliness

Multiple pathways link loneliness to morbidity and mortality, said Cacioppo. Although the deleterious effects of each pathway may be limited, their cumulative effects over time aggregate to produce significant damage to health and well-being. Interventions in these pathways have the potential to mitigate the deleterious effects of loneliness. She identified multiple pathways related to loneliness (Cacioppo and Cacioppo, 2018b; see Table 6-1). Loneliness causes, not just correlates with, increases in vascular resistance and blood pressure. When controlling for all standard predictors or stressors, loneliness can predict blood pressure increases in both older and younger adults (Hawkley et al., 2010b). Loneliness decreases sleep quality through micro-awakenings and poor sleep efficiency (Cacioppo et al., 2002a) and is associated with large increases in the hypothalamic–pituitary–adrenal (HPA) axis stress response; it can predict not only cortisone levels, but cortisone levels the next day (Adam et al., 2006).

Loneliness is associated with increases in depressive symptomatology[1] as well as in prepotent responding, or impassivity. People who feel lonely

[1] Loneliness is a different construct than depression: a person who is lonely feels not only sad, but in danger. Animal studies demonstrate that animals separated from their significant other for at least 2 weeks start showing signs of depressive symptomatology as well.

**TABLE 6-1** Pathways Associated with Loneliness in Human and Animal Models

| Human Experimental and/or Longitudinal Research | Animal Models |
|---|---|
| Increased mortality (Luo et al., 2012) | Increased mortality (Karelina et al., 2009) |
| Increased sleep fragmentation (Cacioppo et al., 2002b; Hawkley et al., 2010a) | Decreased slow wave sleep and homeostatic rebound (Kaushal et al., 2012) |
| Elevated activation of the hypothalamic–pituitary–adrenocortical axis (Adam et al., 2006) | Elevated activation of the hypothalamic–pituitary–adrenocortical axis (Sapolsky et al., 1997) |
| Elevated vascular resistance and blood pressure (Hawkley et al., 2010b) | Elevated blood pressure (Coelho et al., 1991) |
| Up-regulation of gene expression for inflammatory biology and down-regulation of antiviral gene expression (Cole et al., 2007, 2011, 2015) | Up-regulation of gene expression for inflammatory biology and down-regulation of antiviral gene expression (Cole et al., 2015) |
| Decreased viral immunity (Pressman et al., 2005) | Decreased viral immunity (Cole et al., 2015) |
| Increased inflammation (e.g., peripheral IL-6 and IL-beta) (Jaremka et al., 2013) | Increased peripheral inflammation (e.g., peripheral IL-6) (Karelina et al., 2009) |
| Increased impulsive responding, hostility, and defensiveness | Increased prepotent responding and increased aggressiveness (Grippo et al., 2014; Matsumoto et al., 2012; Nin et al., 2011) |
| Increased depression, anxiety, and social withdrawal (Cacioppo et al., 2010) | Increased depression, anxiety, and social withdrawal (Matsumoto et al., 2012; Nin et al., 2011) |

NOTE: IL = interleukin.
SOURCE: Adapted from table presented by Stephanie Cacioppo at the workshop Brain Health Across the Life Span on September 25, 2019.

tend to gamble more, drink more, and consume more fat every day. In line with this impassivity, loneliness also increases suicide rates and ideation. Loneliness also increases defensiveness and self-centeredness. fMRI studies suggest that the latter is mostly due to self-preservation mechanisms and self-survival principles (Cacioppo et al., 2009).[2] Lonely individuals tend to show deactivations of the reward systems in response to positive social versus positive nonsocial stimuli (Aron et al., 2005; Rilling et al., 2002).

[2] Lonely individuals showed hyperactivation of the visual cortex in response to negative social stimuli versus nonsocial stimuli, as well as hyperactivations of temporoparietal junctions on both sides of the brain.

## Brain Dynamics of Loneliness

Cacioppo presented data from studies on the brain dynamics of loneliness that looked at when and how fast the associated brain regions are activated (Cacioppo et al., 2015a, 2016). For example, lonely participants were able to differentiate a social threat from a nonsocial threat about twice as fast as nonlonely participants. Converging evidence suggests that the brain network for alertness is hyperconnected in lonely individuals based on connectivity analysis of resting-state fMRI data. In lonely individuals, investigators observed hyperactivation in the network of alertness (the cingulo-opercular network) and hyperconnectedness in the supramarginal gyrus network, which is associated with taking perspective of other relationships.

Together, the behavioral, neuroimaging, and electroencephalographic (EEG) data suggest that there is a paradoxical element to loneliness. Lonely people feel isolated and receive the biological signal that they need to approach and connect with others to survive. They have this huge motivation to connect, but at the same time, their brains are hyperalert for potential threats to the extent that they see more foes than friends. They tend to see more cues confirming their hypothesis, such as misinterpreted facial expressions of people they are interacting with, then behavioral confirmation processes lead to social withdrawal. Going forward, the temporal dynamics for the operation of loneliness and for each specific pathway need to be better understood. Another research question is to look at whether loneliness is associated with many or all of those pathways in everyone, or if it is associated with different pathways or subsets of pathways across people and social contexts.

## Discussion

Lis Nielsen, chief of the Individual Behavioral Processes Branch of the Division of Behavioral and Social Research at the National Institute on Aging (NIA), remarked that research on loneliness is garnering increased public attention and asked about the level of evidence that would be needed to investigate loneliness targets experimentally. Cacioppo replied that according to an analysis of existing loneliness interventions, one-way social support does not necessarily help as much as other interventions. This is in line with social evolutionary theories that survival depends on mutual aid and protection that is a two-way street of exchanging information and support. Group interventions that bring together people who are lonely are also not very effective owing to the paradox of loneliness. Participants want to go to the meetings, but when they do, they find foes rather than friends. They misinterpret what people are saying, they feel defensiveness, and then they play the blame game. Participants often return home even more distressed because they found confirmation in the behaviors of others. This could be compounded by the tendency of depressed or lonely individuals to remember more negative memories than positive ones, she added. Cognitive behavioral therapeutic interventions tend to be more oriented toward addressing the functions of the social brain network.

Deanna Barch, chair and professor of psychological and brain sciences, professor of radiology, and Gregory B. Couch Professor of Psychiatry at Washington University in St. Louis, asked Cacioppo to elaborate on the nature of loneliness—for example, whether it is a trait-level characteristic. Cacioppo said that we all have the potential to feel lonely at some point in time. It is not an on-off symptom, but a modulation of certain brain areas depending on mind state or mood. Neurotic people tend to be less responsive to some loneliness interventions and less open to being helped with their loneliness. However, she suggested that loneliness is more like a state than a trait, given that a person can go in and out of it so easily.

Damien Fair, associate professor of behavioral neuroscience, associate professor of psychiatry, and associate scientist at the Advanced Imaging Research Center at the Oregon Health & Science University, commented that it is difficult to define brain health without having a target outcome. He suggested that some of the factors Cacioppo discussed in the context of loneliness might be potential targets for brain health writ large, such as quality of life, life expectancy, and the development of psychopathologies. After defining loneliness as a risk factor, the researchers identified brain changes in the animal models, cortisol changes, and behavioral changes related to this risk factor. Fair suggested that the next question is to differentiate between (1) the changes that are related specifically to loneliness or causative of loneliness, and (2) the changes that make one resilient to the risk factor of loneliness. Cacioppo said that longitudinal studies have controlled for the other factors, including genetic expressions, and found that sensitivity to social rejection (not loneliness per se) is heritable 30–35 percent of the time. This sensitivity can be a trigger to all of the other factors. Evidence also shows that constellations of factors like cortisol, sleep salubrity, and the HPA axis drive increases in the effect of loneliness.

Fair asked about individual-level variability in measuring a target such as loneliness, particularly in the temporal domain for prediction purposes. Cacioppo responded that chronic loneliness lasts for at least 2 to 4 weeks; studies should be conducted to understand the individual-level dynamics of loneliness at play during this period. She remarked that loneliness does not discriminate—it touches every gender, every ethnicity, and every context. It has been posited that there are three different types of connections in an individual: intimate connections, relational connections, and collective connections. Further study is warranted to understand the relationships between those connections (or lack thereof) and loneliness. Early research suggests that the collective connections do not move as fast as the intimate ones or the relational ones; collective connections tend to be protective of personal loneliness. Cacioppo said:

> If you have a sense that you belong to someone even if you feel lonely every other day, the fact that you belong to a group that is bigger than yourself—and you have a bigger purpose in life—that would be really helpful for you to feel less lonely on a daily basis.

## MOTIVATION, COGNITION, AND DECISION MAKING IN EVERYDAY LIFE

Samanez-Larkin focused on potential ways that emotional health actually improves with age. Attention is often focused on the relatively linear declines associated with aging in terms of fluid cognitive deficits, attention, inhibiting interference, memory, and so forth. However, evidence that older adults experience more positive emotions and fewer negative emotions in daily life—and report being better able to control their emotions—suggest that emotional health may improve with age in some respects.

Longitudinal evidence from positron emission tomography (PET) and fMRI studies provides insight into the functional and structural changes in the brain that account for age-related impairments in cognition. For example, this evidence suggests that changes in episodic memory, which would typically be ascribed to the medial temporal lobes, seem to be related more strongly to gradual structural and functional decline causing gross losses in the frontal cortex. However, the neurobiological bases of motivational and emotional health improvements are not yet well understood. Even today, some researchers maintain a dualistic position with respect to biology and motivation—meaning, that findings about age differences in cognition are either attributable to biological changes or to motivational changes, as if motivational changes are not biological. This highlights the need for research on how motivational systems may change with age in ways that maintain the stability of emotional health and may even drive improvements.

### Neurobiology of Age Differences in Decision Making

To help address this research gap, Samanez-Larkin's group looks at how individual and age differences in motivation and cognition influence decision making across the life span. Decision making is a capacity that recruits a broad range of interacting psychological processes and neurobiological systems. Their early research found that older adults tend to perform the same or better as younger adults in some decision tasks—such as intertemporal choice tasks—but they tend to perform worse than younger adults in certain types of tasks, such as reinforcement learning.[3] He noted that the older adults still learned in these tasks, it just took more time.

Reinforcement learning tasks require learning quickly from experience. Early fMRI studies suggested that the age difference in reinforcement learning tasks was related, at least in part, to reduced representation of prediction errors in the medial prefrontal cortex in older adults. He described this as a weaker teaching signal in the ventral medial prefrontal regions. These brain regions contain many dopamine receptors, so it was assumed that this age-related difference in decision making was likely related to a dopaminergic deficit with age. In fact, subsequent studies showed that giving participants the dopamine precursor levodopa could improve reinforcement learning in older adults and normalize that value-based signal in the prefrontal cortex. This highlights the important role of dopamine in reinforcement learning and suggests that declines in reinforcement learning are caused by decreasing levels of dopamine with age.

Neuroimaging evidence also sheds some light on why older adults seem to perform the same, if not better, on decision-making tasks involving intertemporal choice. In some studies, older adults were more likely to wait for a larger reward than younger adults, who tended to choose a smaller reward that was immediately available. Evidence from fMRI studies shows that older people were primarily representing the reward magnitude in the medial prefrontal cortex. This suggests that the older adults were less likely to factor the delay into their decision making and that the value signal seen in older adults is mostly a function of the reward's magnitude; behaviorally, the time delay does not appear to matter as much. Evidence from different laboratories showed the same pattern, with the clusters associated with age differences occurring in almost exactly the same places, but the researchers' conclusions based on those similar findings were very different.

Samanez-Larkin's group maintained that the findings are evidence for preservation with age. They speculated that older adults have more lived experience and thus understand that a delayed large reward will feel just as good or better than an immediate small reward. Another research group came to the opposite conclusion, that these findings are evidence for decline with age. They suggested that older adults have a motivational deficit in that they cannot muster as much excitement

[3] Typically, reinforcement learning tasks requiring the participant to make a choice, receive feedback, and then make a new choice based on the evidence provided thus far.

about an early or immediate reward as younger people can, which is likely related to reduced motivational dopaminergic signaling in older adults. Samanez-Larkin's group hypothesized that older adults tend to perform worse on reinforcement learning tasks and the same or better on choice-based decision tasks for the same reason: they are more willing to tolerate delays due to decline of dopamine with age and a consequent global motivational deficit. In other words, older people find it harder to get excited and motivated. This hypothesis is counter to findings about emotional experience and age-related social preferences conducted by Carstensen and other social-psychology-oriented aging labs, which suggest that motivation changes with age, but it does not go away.

### Time Horizons and Goals Shift with Age

Socioemotional selectivity theory holds that time horizons change with age. As people age, the awareness that time is limited influences their goals and changes their motivation. Some of the early evidence about age-related changes in motivation came from simple social partner preference studies, in which participants are asked to choose a person with whom to spend 30 minutes of free time—with the author of a book the person recently read, with a recent acquaintance with whom the person seems to have much in common, or with a close friend or family member (Carstensen and Fredrickson, 1998; Fredrickson and Carstensen, 1990; Fung et al., 1999).

Younger people are more likely to choose the author or recent acquaintance and are somewhat indifferent in their preference for the three options. Older adults tend to be less indifferent than younger people and demonstrate a strong preference for the close social partner, who is associated with known usefulness and positive value. Based on this evidence, investigators hypothesized that the age effects on behavior, and potentially on brain function, depend on the goal relevance of the rewards. The early work on reward processing in the aging brain from his lab had used monetary rewards, so it is possible that the older adult participants tended to be more financially comfortable, making the small monetary reward less motivating.

Samanez-Larkin's group has explored age-related differences in how the type of reward relates to motivation. One study hypothesized that age effects on behavior and frontostriatal function would depend on the goal relevance of rewards. The study used three versions of the intertemporal choice task (Seaman et al., 2016): (1) a standard version of the task, in which participants chose between an immediate smaller monetary reward and a delayed larger monetary reward; (2) a social version of the task, in which the reward magnitude was the length of time spent with a close social partner; and (3) a health version of the task, in which the reward magnitude was the dosage of a hypothetical drug that would improve organ function as well as cognitive and mental health. Figure 6-1 shows that in the monetary reward task, older people are statistically as likely to choose the immediate option as younger people. However, in the social and health reward tasks, older adults are more likely to take the smaller immediate reward than younger people.[4]

These findings warrant a behavioral explanation, because if low dopamine levels reduce the motivation for immediate reward in older people, they can apparently still become excited for immediate rewards behaviorally. Another study looked at subjective value signals during three decision-making tasks.

Each participant's individual preferences were taken into account based on their behavioral choices, in order to look at the representation of subjective usefulness and subjective value. In this study, age differences were not observed in the medial prefrontal cortex; the adults of all ages similarly represented subjective value. This suggests that this basic value signal or usefulness signal in the brain seems to be stable across adulthood (Seaman et al., 2018).

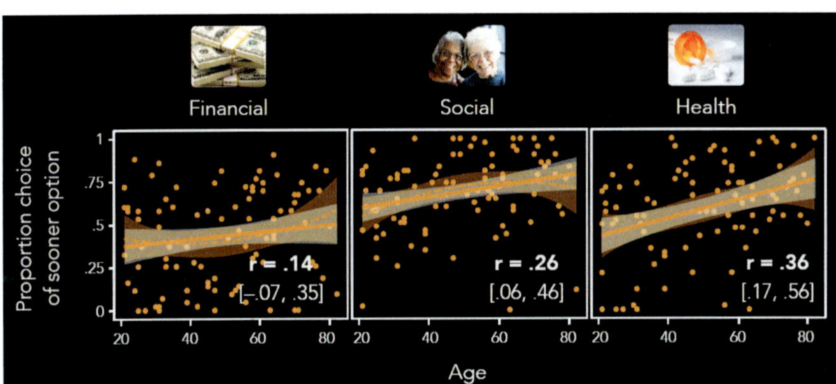


**FIGURE 6-1** Older adults want immediate social and health rewards.
SOURCES: As presented by Gregory Samanez-Larkin at the workshop Brain Health Across the Life Span on September 25, 2019; adapted from Seaman et al., 2016.

[4] Samanez-Larkin noted that in other studies, the positive effect is generally not seen in the financial reward task. He posited that because the financial, social, and health tasks were intermixed in this study, perhaps it oriented the older adults' future thinking in such a way that they are more focused on the present in the financial task than they might normally be.

## Age Differences in the Dopamine System

To further investigate the functional sequelae of the well-established, age-related dopamine decline, Samanez-Larkin's group conducted a meta-analysis of different components of the dopamine system. After analyzing three decades of PET and single-photon emission computed tomography (SPECT) imaging studies of adult age differences in the dopamine system, researchers found very strong declines in dopamine transporters across both classes of dopamine receptors (i.e., D1-like and D2-like receptors). However, they did not find significant age difference in dopamine synthesis capacity, which is a measure of how well dopamine can be packaged and prepared for release (Karrer et al., 2017). This suggests that older adults are able to produce dopamine and package it relatively well, but the receptor differences limit the extent to which that dopamine can affect signaling. Signal transmission may be limited because there are fewer sites to act postsynaptically. The age-related decline in dopamine transporters may actually be helpful, he noted, because the transporters are located on the presynaptic cells that pull dopamine back in. When there are fewer transporters, there is more dopamine present that can potentially act postsynaptically.

## Evidence for Motivational Brain Health

This evidence for the health of the aging dopamine system was interesting, but the underlying processes were still unclear, given the very strong age correlations with D2-like and D1-like receptors. The researchers posited that perhaps the motivational effects and functional value signals in the medial prefrontal cortex—a brain region that has significantly more glutamate than dopamine receptors—functionally shift away from the dopamine system as people age. In the meta-analysis, the reported statistics yielded very large regions of interest, including the prefrontal cortex and all of the striatum. To address this, Samanez-Larkin's group used higher-resolution data from 132 adults ranging in age from 20 to 85 years to look more closely at the striatum and certain cortical regions (Seaman et al., 2019). They parsed up frontal cortex into all the sub gyri, the striatum into all the striatal subregions, and the mediotemporal lobe into subregions, and then plotted the percentage differences per decade in D2-like-receptor availability. The analysis showed substantial regional variation in the decline of D2-like receptors with aging (see Figure 6-2). Certain regions show a strong percentage decline per decade estimated from these cross-sectional data, while other regions show no evidence of an age effect.[5] The strongest declines were seen in the lateral frontal

[5] All of the data are available at http://bit.ly/agingdopamine (accessed November 13, 2019).

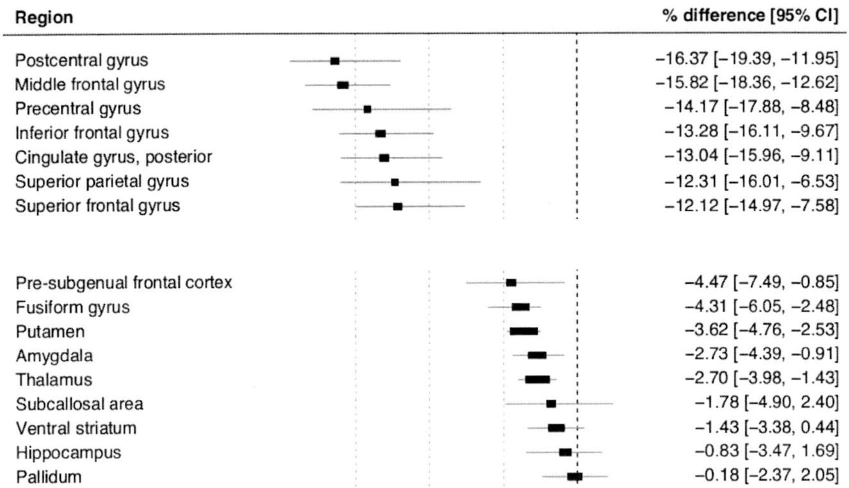


**FIGURE 6-2** Regional variation in the decline of D2-like receptors with aging.
NOTE: CI = confidence interval.
SOURCES: As presented by Gregory Samanez-Larkin at the workshop Brain Health Across the Life Span on September 25, 2019; adapted from Seaman et al., 2019.

cortex, while the weakest effects (or no effects) were seen in the ventral striatum and pallidum.

Samanez-Larkin emphasized that this evidence does not support the idea of global motivational decline. Even though the declines in the dopamine system are well documented, the meta-analysis revealed that synthesis capacities are relatively preserved; D2-like receptors are also preserved in certain regions of the brain. It appears that dopamine production, postsynaptic action, and signal transmission are maintained with age in certain subcomponents of these circuits. Perhaps some subparts of the circuits are actually working relatively well and their functions are dopamine mediated, which would affect fMRI evidence for preserved signaling. This could also be caused by the preservation of dopamine in those circuits. He suggested that evidence for motivational brain health—rather than decline—is the meaningful evidence that is emerging from this fMRI, behavioral, and PET research.

### Future Research Directions

Samanez-Larkin concluded by describing some of his laboratory's future research directions. They have ongoing fMRI studies on anticipation and the experience of social versus health rewards, as well as plans for PET studies to look at how different types of rewards elicit dopamine release in different parts of the dopamine system as people age. Although his team is using somewhat more naturalistic stimuli, the paradigms are still relatively basic—positive social rewards, negative social rewards, or social incentives (Holland et al., 2019). They are also looking at how these reward-type differences influence function, as well as how those factors are related to differences in dopamine levels.

## Discussion

Barch asked about age-related changes in neurotransmitter systems other than dopamine. Samanez-Larkin replied that his laboratory recently completed a meta-analysis on the age effects of serotonin; there appears to be no preservation of the serotonin system and a relatively clear decline with age. Nielsen asked if there is any evidence that individual differences in the dopamine system are a function of life-course individual differences in impulsivity or other traits, or any evidence about individual differences in loneliness or social isolation in terms of the response to social reward tasks. Samanez-Larkin replied that this type of social engagement information is not collected very well in this arena. In general, however, his group's work shows between-subject variability at every age, with very strong individual differences, even though the age effects are relatively consistent; more work remains to be done to explain that variance.

Fair remarked that two items can cause the type of variance that is seen in these data: one is the real signal—that is, the real variability with regard to a given measurement—and the other is noise. The two may need to be teased apart to understand what it means to be resilient. Samanez-Larkin responded by acknowledging the limitations of these cross-sectional data. Very little longitudinal PET data are available, and some of the changes they are investigating take decades to become apparent. It might be possible to identify lifestyle factors and create retrospective measures, but there is no earlier time point to relate the data to; the participants could simply have wildly different intercepts and the same rates of age-related receptor loss. In terms of noisy data in general, Samanez-Larkin's group is interested in brain signal variability. They have analyzed functional neural signal variability in fMRI data to ascertain how volatile the brain signal is, how that variability changes with age, and how it is related to decision making; they are also looking at whether fMRI signal variability is related to differences in dopamine receptors.

## LIFE-COURSE CAUSES OF LATER-LIFE INEQUALITIES IN BRAIN HEALTH

Manly presented on life-course causes of inequalities and disparities in brain health later in life. She began with a review of challenges faced in researching brain health disparities. First, this research cannot be conducted using convenience samples, which proliferates in research on older adult brain health. The second challenge is that brain health disparities research must measure life-course individual or contextual factors, such as social determinants of health or the social exposome, sufficiently well to determine the relative contributions of bio-psycho-behavioral-social factors to disease or interactions. Experts in quantifying brain health have not traditionally focused on social determinants of health across the life course. As a result, measurements of social determinants are often lacking even in studies that have exquisite measurements of brain health outcomes. This has hampered discovery and acceleration in the field of brain health disparities.

A third challenge is the difficulty in determining the degree of bias in estimates of early-life or life-course factors and how they relate to brain health. Observational research will not have value unless it is used to develop targeted interventions using accurate estimates. However, it is difficult to determine bias if the target or reference population has not been defined, thus threatening external and internal validity. The fourth challenge is to develop harmonized measures,[6] both of risk factors and of brain health outcomes; these are critical for combining cohorts, synthesizing research, and accelerating knowledge.

### Evidence for Disparities in Later-Life Brain Health and Resilience

Manly provided an overview of available evidence for disparities in brain health and in aging, as well as some of the methodological challenges in research and some of the identified mechanisms that could help to explain these disparities in later-life brain health. The Washington Heights–Inwood Columbia Aging Project (WHICAP) longitudinal study in Northern Manhattan found that African Americans and Caribbean Hispanics are more likely to develop incident Alzheimer's disease over time (Tang et al., 2001). These disparities persist even after adjusting for years of education, occupation, income, or history of stroke, hypertension,

[6] Harmonized measures are measures that are standard across research groups and fields. Harmonized measures may avoid the problem of duplicative or overlapping research, as well as allowing larger studies to be conducted with greater power to observe subtle phenomena related to brain health and resilience.

and diabetes. Furthermore, the interventions that would be expected to mediate these differences do not seem to have a substantial effect on these disparities.

Evidence of racial and ethnic disparities was also found in the Kaiser Permanente Health Study in Northern California, which followed people in the health care system over many years. African Americans, American Indians, and Alaskan Natives were found to have the highest risk of developing dementia, while Asian Americans were at lower risk. Although researchers were not able to look at some of the social factors, such as education, that might explain these disparities in incident dementia, they were able to look at cerebrovascular and cardiovascular disease, but found that these did not explain the disparities (Mayeda et al., 2016).

Manly noted that there is also a geographic dimension to these disparities in risk for Alzheimer's disease and dementia. An analysis of the Centers for Disease Control and Prevention death records found that both African Americans and whites have a higher risk of dying of all-cause dementia if they were born in a "stroke belt" state; even if they migrated to the north and eventually died there, they brought this risk with them from the South (Glymour et al., 2011). Racial disparities in stroke are well known—with African Americans at higher risk—but it is less commonly known that whites aged 85 years and older are at higher risk of having stroke than African Americans, according to a national longitudinal study of stroke disparities (Howard et al., 2011).

## Methodological Challenges in Brain Health Disparities Research

Manly highlighted the influence of selection bias in this field. The studies she presented in the previous section are population-representative, community-based longitudinal studies. Selection bias is prevalent in studies that use clinic-based or convenience samples, in which participants are recruited from clinics that specialize in memory disorders, for example. Mistrust and stigma are direct causes of the problem of selection bias. She noted that a long history of stigma and mistrust persists to this day, widening the gap between the people who have cognitive impairments and the people who go to a doctor with those complaints. This is a consequence of historical medical abuses, including use of IQ tests to support racist policies, as well as the lack of evidence on the benefits of medical research for underserved communities facing intractable disparities. Ongoing experiences of discrimination in the medical setting are common, and health care systems broadly lack the necessary cultural and linguistic competencies.

The Minority Aging Research Study in Chicago found that African Americans who were diagnosed with clinical Alzheimer's disease dementia were more likely to have mixed neuropathology than whites who had the same diagnosis (Barnes et al., 2015). However, the number of whites that participated in autopsy far exceeds the number of African Americans. Thus, the findings do not necessarily indicate that Alzheimer's disease has more mixed pathology in African Americans versus whites—it is possible that the African Americans who volunteered for the study were more likely to get diagnosed with Alzheimer's disease. African Americans who are formally diagnosed with Alzheimer's disease tend to have more psychiatric symptoms of irritability, agitation, paranoia, and behavioral issues than whites who are formally diagnosed.

The problem of selection bias even affects studies that are looking to characterize neuropathology in vivo. A study that has been recruiting African Americans in St. Louis for cerebrospinal fluid lumbar puncture collection and PET amyloid imaging recently concluded that there are race-dependent biological mechanisms for these expressions of Alzheimer's disease (Morris et al., 2019). Researchers found that the African Americans in their study had less cerebrospinal fluid t-tau. However, the African Americans were matched to the whites in the cohort for years of education, which Manly suggested is not representative of the community in St. Louis or anywhere in the country. Furthermore, the African Americans in their cohort did not have any more cerebrovascular-disease-like white-matter hyperintensities than did the whites in the cohorts, which signals that the African Americans in their study are unusual.

### Potential Mechanisms for Disparities

An analysis of the Midlife in the United States (MIDUS) and WHICAP studies found a narrowing of the disparity in memory performance between African Americans and whites in the older age group. This is evidence for an age-as-leveler effect, said Manly. People from minority groups who survive longer tend to be a heartier cohort than white people who survive into midlife, as a function of survival bias (Zahodne et al., 2016). This survivor effect helps to explain the crossover of stroke prevalence across race as people age that was described in the previous section (Howard et al., 2011).

Another mechanism that has been focused on in explaining brain health disparities is cerebrovascular disease. There are disparities in the burden of white-matter hyperintensities across race (Brickman et al., 2008). Whites have a lower overall burden of white-matter hyperintensities compared to African Americans and Hispanics, with no apparent interaction with age, but the scanning began when people were around 70 years of age. Interaction or acceleration must have occurred at some point earlier among the African Americans and Hispanics. This highlights another challenge: understanding the neuropathological mechanisms underlying brain health disparities will require studying people earlier in life.

A more recent study found a tighter link between white-matter hyperintensity burden and cognition in African Americans than in whites (Zahodne et al., 2015). This contrasts with the same study's findings about the relationship between cognitive trajectory and hippocampal volume. Whites with low hippocampal volume were at higher risk for developing Alzheimer's disease than whites with high hippocampal volume, but hippocampal volume was not related to risk of developing Alzheimer's disease among the non-Hispanic African Americans in the study. This suggests that there may be different pathways to cognitive decline across race and ethnicity.

Many researchers have been looking at genetic research to try to explain some of the disparities in brain health. However, these ancestry differences can generally be explained by social factors. One study compared African Americans with Alzheimer's disease to matched controls, finding that higher levels of African ancestry (both at the whole genome level and at specific Alzheimer's disease–related genetic loci, like ABCA7) are associated with an increased risk for Alzheimer's disease (Hohman et al., 2016). However, Manly cautioned that social factors correlate with African ancestry and could confound the relationships with cognitive outcomes—in other words, African ancestry may be a very strong marker for experiences of discrimination and other social factors. Higher African ancestry has been associated with having a lower education level, having parents with fewer years of schooling, receiving no inheritance from one's parents, having a lower income, and having less wealth. Ancestry does not biologically mediate or influence these factors, but African ancestry is a marker for social experiences of individuals, parents, and grandparents. In other diseases associated with genetic ancestral markers, such as diabetes, these types of social factors account for the relationship between ancestry and disease (Marden et al., 2016).

Manly's group is working on a study based on the WHICAP cohort dataset looking at cognitive outcomes, racial self-identification, and African ancestry among Caribbean Latino older adults who were followed longitudinally.[7] Those people in the lowest quartile of African ancestry had higher cognitive test scores compared to people with a higher degree of African ancestry, but these differences are explained entirely by the quality and quantity of the person's educational experience and by the

[7] Available at http://www.nationalacademies.org/hmd/Activities/Aging/BrainHealthAcrossTheLifeSpanWorkshop/2019-JUN-26.aspx (accessed March 12, 2020).

person's early-life socioeconomic status, which is mainly driven by the degree of the person's education.

## Forthcoming Research on Brain Health Disparities

Manly described forthcoming research based on the dataset from the ongoing Reasons for Geographic and Racial Differences in Stroke (REGARDS) study, which has followed a large and geographically diverse cohort of older adults in the United States to look at vascular contributions to cognitive impairment and dementia. An advantage of the REGARDS dataset is that it collects data about every place each participant has ever lived.

### *Effect of Historical Investments in Quality of Schooling on Cognition Later in Life*

Economists have been using the administrative data from schools for many years to predict human capital outcomes and show differences across race in those outcomes. Manly's group used administrative data to explore the relationship between school quality and race across time and location. Specifically, they looked at the effect of historical investments in quality of schooling on cognition later in life. For instance, the length of the academic year for schools in the South, particularly for those with African American students, was much shorter than in the North. If an African American person born in the 1930s reports having gone to school for 8 years in certain states, it is likely that the school was only open about half of the year. Similarly, the student–teacher ratio for African American children in some states was very high, which has an effect on later-life cognition. After controlling for early-life confounds, such as family socioeconomic status, as well as for state-level or state-fixed effects, Manly's team found that people across races who attended schools with longer term lengths had improved cognition compared to people who attended schools in states or counties that had shorter term lengths.[8]

Based on these data, Manly's team developed an overall score for school quality based on these administrative records. For every 1-year increase of policy-predicted years of education, people in the REGARDS study were at 40 percent lower odds of having cognitive impairment at baseline. Adding confounds such as age, sex, gender, state fixed effects, and parent education reveals an interaction in which white women, white

[8] Manly, J. Workshop presentation—Life-Course Causes of Later-Life Inequalities in Brain Health. Available at http://www.nationalacademies.org/hmd/Activities/Aging/BrainHealthAcrossTheLifeSpanWorkshop/2019-JUN-26.aspx (accessed March 12, 2020).

men, and African American women have a payoff for going to higher-quality schools, but not African American men.

*Discrimination and Cognitive Function Among Older Non-Hispanic African Americans*

Manly's group is also working on studies of discrimination and cognitive function. Preliminary findings suggest that in general, African Americans with more education report experiencing more discrimination. Furthermore, there is interaction between sex, years of education, and discrimination on cognitive function. The trend is that self-reported discrimination among African American men with graduate degrees is negatively related to cognition; this is not the case for African American men who have high school or college degrees.

*Leveraging Expanded Datasets*

Moving the field of disparities in brain health forward will require taking advantage of studies that start at an earlier age, said Manly. Her group has identified a number of cohorts that began when participants were in high school, such as the Project TALENT dataset and the High School and Beyond dataset. These studies conducted cognitive testing when participants were adolescents, which allows for tracking survival (and potentially for the survival effect) as well as for looking at early-life predictors of later-life cognition. Project TALENT is being linked to Medicare, which has been used to show that lower levels of cognitive function as an adolescent predicted a formal diagnosis of Alzheimer's disease later in life (Huang et al., 2018).

## Ways Forward to Improve Research on Brain Health Disparities

Manly concluded by offering strategies for improving research on brain health disparities going forward. Racism should be measured in Alzheimer's disease and related dementia studies, because systemic racism becomes embodied in the biology of racialized groups. This is how race becomes a risk factor for later-life problems or inequalities in brain health. Measuring racism will require designing population-based longitudinal studies that bridge the gap between (1) biology and genetics and (2) the life course and social exposome. Population-feasible biomarkers for neuropathology will need to be developed and included in these studies; lumbar puncture or PET will not be feasible, so blood tests will probably need to be developed in diverse cohorts. Only with all of those factors measured in the same cohort will it be possible to calculate population-attributable factors. This would allow researchers to explore how intervening in certain social factors could have an effect across the life course.

Regardless of their size, highly selected samples are not useful for disparities research (Keyes and Westreich, 2019). Researchers looking at brain health disparities need more clarity about the limits of convenience or volunteer samples, how to control for the confounds of sampling, and how to discuss these confounds in their work. Social forces such as racism and discrimination, educational quality and increasing school segregation, and neighborhood inequalities should be acknowledged explicitly in national plans to reduce the effect or burden of neuropathology and Alzheimer's disease and related dementia on the population. Doing so will require unequivocally making the case that early-life economic and social policy is tantamount to brain health policy, perhaps through Alzheimer's disease national plans, Alzheimer's disease summits, and accountability measures.

## Discussion

Bruce McEwen, Alfred E. Mirsky Professor at The Rockefeller University, remarked that the Safe American Family (SAF) study has looked at how building bonds between adolescents and their parents or caregivers, as well as mitigating bullying and racial discrimination, can improve physical and mental health outcomes 10 to 15 years later, including brain volume and type 2 diabetes. Manly replied that it is critical to understand how these types of interventions have effects throughout the life course; the role of inflammation in metabolic syndromes and Alzheimer's disease, for example, warrants further investigation. McEwen added that insulin resistance is a known pathway toward dementia that can be exacerbated—especially in people with certain genotypes—by experiences such as abuse, neglect, and poverty. Understanding the roles of inflammation and overactivity of glutamatergic systems in the brain that drive the amyloid-beta hypothesis about Alzheimer's disease could be further enriched by studying attempts to intervene early, as in the SAF study.

Lis Nielsen asked about how to enhance the value of datasets for studying health disparities, for example, by adding retrospective measures of social exposome variables to studies that focused on older age or by designing earlier life-course studies to incorporate those types of measures, so they will be valuable for long-term studies of aging and brain health. In terms of retrospective measures that could be added, Manly emphasized the value of retrospectively collecting and geocoding location data from older adult participants about every place they have ever lived. These data have great value in analyzing the effects of childhood exposures and administrative policies in educational systems on the trajectory of brain health. For example, they can be used to look at factors such as walkability, green spaces, business, and crime.

Studies are looking at how the policing and punishment policies in individual schools may relate to stress and outcomes in children as well as to later-life outcomes. In terms of designing early-life studies to add value to later-life research, Manly suggested that cognitive function is important for understanding the real effects of interventions. At the age of 65 years, a person is at an intercept that is strongly related to family history, young life cognition, and exposures after that age. Much research on Alzheimer's disease and related dementias is focused on slope, distinguishing the trajectories with respect to slope over time, and its relationship to hippocampal volume, diabetes, and other biomarkers. The biggest effect to be had in maintaining brain health is on the intercept with which a person enters older age. Thus, early-life studies and measures of cognition earlier in life are critical for determining the potential effect of interventions.

## PANEL DISCUSSION ON BRAIN HEALTH IN THE SOCIAL CONTEXT

Fair asked the panelists to discuss how the definition of brain health affects how its outcomes should be measured—for instance, quality of life and stress are reflected in various types of outcomes depending on the population being described. Barch replied that brain health can be thought about as (1) a person's accumulative reserve, which sets the intercept or starting point, and (2) the degree to which a person is affected by adversities, such as stress or the onset of illness. These adversities are likely to be related and difficult to tease apart unless they are measured from an early stage—from birth or even in utero would be ideal. Social determinants are being set in utero, and exposures could potentially be setting up a proinflammatory phenotype very early in life that has effects later. More practically, it would be helpful to focus on intermediate outcomes that are already known to be predictive and to look at whether their genesis is even earlier than assumed.

Manly suggested that in the context of aging brain health, it would be useful to be explicit that the trajectories of cognitive decline start much earlier in life, before they have their greatest effect on function and impose the greatest burden and cost to society. Manly also highlighted the challenge of how to measure brain health across the entire life course. She suggested linking and triangulating among studies focusing on different time periods during the life course. Even if the studies do not use the same cognitive measures or focus on the same outcomes, this strategy may be useful as a starting point for exploring potential targets and identifying critical periods across the life course. Fair noted the importance of bringing context to bear in prospectively trying to coordinate and design new studies and new research. Ted Satterthwaite, assistant professor in the Department of Psychiatry at the University of Pennsylvania School of Medicine, remarked that investment will be needed to harmonize, chain back, and link those data sources. A relatively small, inexpensive study could harmonize different measures and outcomes across large-scale expensive studies, so they can be linked in different populations of interest and provide additional return on that investment.

# 7

# Brain Health Across the Life Span

**Key Points Highlighted by Workshop Participants**

- Standardized psychiatric interviews include hundreds of questions about symptoms, but most psychiatric imaging studies take a very reduced look at these data. Although this approach is reasonable, it is based on the assumption—which is not well supported by evidence—that the biological scale of the abnormalities matches with the scale of data reduction. Another alternative is to try to directly integrate high-dimensional brain data. (Ted Satterthwaite)
- Electronic health records are already capturing important biologically based measures that could be easily scaled—through mobile platforms or otherwise—and then linked to meaningful health outcomes. Currently, differential treatment response to measures of brain health is a major gap in the literature that will need to be addressed to make this research clinically actionable. Building systems of informatics could also help to link biological measures to health outcomes. (Ted Satterthwaite)
- There is a range of commonsense good practices that can improve brain health, such as exercise and sleep. However,

this does not imply that these practices will prevent the occurrence of Alzheimer's disease or other brain disorders with underlying genetic factors. (Deanna Barch)

- There is evidence that individuals with a history of early life adversity may be differentially responsive to treatments for depression and other mental disorders, but clinics do not typically ask about those factors. There may be value in collecting such data to examine implications for preventive and treatment interventions addressing a range of cognitive and emotional disorders. (Lis Nielsen)

This chapter focuses on brain health throughout the life span, with respect to typical brain development as well as the development of psychiatric disorders. The session explored how brain health and resilience change across the life span and how researchers have measured these changes. Presenters and panelists also discussed the signals that changes in vulnerabilities and opportunities can provide about brain health and resilience at various life stages. An overview of early adversity, emotional processing, and the neural bases of psychiatric illness was provided by Deanna Barch, chair and professor of psychological and brain sciences, professor of radiology, and Gregory B. Couch Professor of Psychiatry at Washington University in St. Louis. Nim Tottenham, professor in the Department of Psychology at Columbia University, looked at the effect of early-life stress on neurodevelopment. Ted Satterthwaite, assistant professor in the Department of Psychiatry at the University of Pennsylvania School of Medicine, examined how the integration of complex and personalized data can be used to understand normal and abnormal brain network development. Brain network aging and health across the adult life span was described by Gagan Wig, associate professor of behavioral and brain sciences at the Center for Vital Longevity at the University of Texas at Dallas.

## EARLY ADVERSITY, EMOTIONAL PROCESSING, AND THE NEURAL BASES OF PSYCHIATRIC ILLNESS

Barch's presentation explored sensitive periods in which environmental influences have particularly strong relationships to brain health. Studying how these influences affect mental health later in life can shed light on the temporality of those influences—meaning, how early in the process of brain development they have an effect. Many of the factors that appear to be critical seem to be emerging earlier and earlier, she noted, which underlines the importance of investigating neonatal maternal health. Environmental factors that are not consistent with the expected input at specific developmental stages—such as lack of parental support early in life—might be most detrimental to brain health (Gabard-Durnam and McLaughlin, 2019). Similarly, the presence of input that should not be happening at a given time, owing to various types of adversity, may also be very damaging at certain periods of life. This likely interacts with what is happening in the brain during these periods. Myelination and experience-dependent processes, such as pruning,[1] can vary by brain region. This suggests that there is developmental specificity to the effects of adversity and nurturance on mental health; these effects vary by region and may be differently susceptible at various points in development. Understanding these differences can guide decisions about when to intervene for optimal success.

## Maternal Support and Brain Development

Barch focused on maternal support and brain development, with the caveat that paternal support is also important, but good quality measures of paternal support are very limited. A rich body of literature from rodent and nonhuman primate studies clearly demonstrates that the presence of a nurturing caregiver early in life has a powerful effect on hippocampal development and function. This occurs through epigenetic mechanisms that are modulated by various aspects of early caregiving (Fish et al., 2004; Liu et al., 1997; Meaney, 2001; Szyf et al., 2005). Animal models have been able to elucidate some of the causal effects of maternal support because investigators are able to experimentally manipulate this variable.

Carrying out similar research in humans is challenging, because the factors that drive the presence or absence of maternal support could also be contributing to brain development in children through genetic processes or other factors that are difficult to tease apart. However, available data in humans are consistent with the animal study data in suggesting that early experiences of maternal support—or conversely, of abuse, neglect, or adversity—also affect human hippocampal development (Bremner et al., 1997; Driessen et al., 2000; Stein et al., 1997). The hippocampus is a structure that is dense with glucocorticoid receptors and is important in stress regulation and stress modulation through its integral role in the hypothalamic–pituitary–adrenal axis stress response. It has been suggested that reductions and disruptions to hippocampal volume and function lead to maladaptive stress reactivity later in life, which makes it more difficult for a child to engage in appropriate emotion

[1] A normal developmental process in which the connections between neurons are reduced.

regulation and coping. Later in life, this can contribute to affective psychopathologies such as depression and anxiety (Luby et al., 2016).

### Effect of Preschool Maternal Support on the Trajectory of Hippocampal Volume

In humans, it is not yet clear whether there are "sensitive" periods during which parental nurturance to brain development is either more or less important. To explore this question, Barch described a long-term longitudinal study that recruited a sample of around 300 preschoolers between the ages of 3 and 5 years that began in 2002 and is still going on today (Luby et al., 2016). Each year, the participants receive intensive assessments of psychopathology, home factors, and observational, objectively coded measures of structured maternal support and parent–child interaction. Longitudinal neuroimaging began when the children were 7 or 8 years of age (it is currently in its fifth wave), and investigators are still following the participants using a wide range of behavioral assessments.

Neuroimaging data were used to look at the trajectories of hippocampal development in the participants between the ages of roughly 7 and 16 years. A multilevel linear model allows for looking at the entire trajectory of hippocampal volume development across multiple waves, while controlling for factors such as whole-brain gray matter. The investigators also looked at whether the measures of preschool maternal support and school-age maternal support have main effects (i.e., overall hippocampal volume) or interactions over time. The latter are interactions with changes in hippocampal volume over time as children grow. In the preschool age range, they found an upward slope typical of hippocampal volume development in the growth period. The only effect that holds is that of preschool maternal support on the slope of hippocampal volume, which positively predicts children's self-report management of sad emotions. The greater the preschool maternal support, the steeper the increase in hippocampal volume development over time (see Figure 7-1). This suggests that preschool is a sensitive period for the influence of maternal support on the trajectory of hippocampal development.

The findings for the longitudinal preschool study are consistent with the animal literature suggesting that early maternal support has a positive effect on hippocampal structure and function.[2] The importance of larger hippocampal volume to emotional regulation was demonstrated when

---

[2] Barch noted that animal models typically do not measure hippocampal volume; they tend to measure more molecular and cellular processes related to hippocampal development—so the human and animal study results do not mirror each other exactly, but they are consistent.

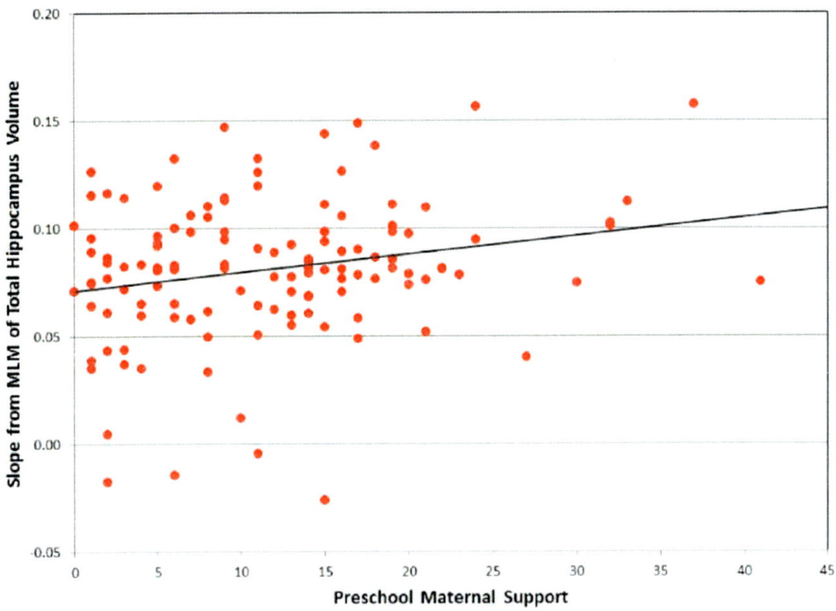


**FIGURE 7-1** Individually estimated slopes over time for total hippocampus volume as a function of preschool maternal support.
NOTE: MLM = multilevel linear model.
SOURCES: As presented by Deanna Barch at the workshop Brain Health Across the Life Span on September 25, 2019; Luby et al., 2016.

the study participants were in mid-adolescence. The participants with the steepest upward growth of hippocampal volume reported being the most effective at managing their negative emotions. This relationship was supported by both the self-reported and the parent-reported measures of emotion regulation. Steeper hippocampal volume growth was also associated with better episodic memory function in later adolescence.

### Adverse Childhood Experiences and Interactions with Maternal Support

The outcome of the trajectory of hippocampal growth on later behaviors can be tied to early maternal support effects, said Barch. Although maternal support is important, many other adversities can occur during early childhood. In theory, these types of adverse childhood experiences (ACEs) could be connected to maternal support; for example, maternal support could be affected by parental psychopathology, also producing an ACE. However, other ACEs are relatively independent of parental behavior, such as poverty and exposure to trauma not perpetrated by parents. Research on the effect of ACEs on child development has generated good data that early childhood adversity also relates to the structural and functional development of limbic regions including the hippocampus, the amygdala, the basal ganglia, and cortical regions (Carrión et al., 2010; Edmiston et al., 2011; Hanson et al., 2015; McDermott et al., 2019; Rao et al., 2010).

More information is needed on the potentially interactive effects of early childhood adversity and caregiver support, as well as the developmental timing in which these two things have their strongest relationships to brain outcomes. Some evidence suggests that maternal support may have protective effects for children, in the sense that children may be buffered from some of the effects of nonmaternal-related ACEs by having strong maternal support. This could be attributable to a resilience factor, but it could also be the result of the additive contributions that maternal support provides to a child's brain health and development.[3]

In recent work, Barch and colleagues analyzed data from a longitudinal study to look for independent or interactive effects of maternal support and ACEs on brain development in preschool- and school-aged children. In this study, they looked at the hippocampus but also looked more broadly at various subcortical and cortical brain regions, including the hippocampus, the amygdala, the subgenual cingulate cortex, and the caudate. Maternal support was assessed using the measure described in the previous section. ACEs were defined as poverty (defined as an income-to-needs ratio of less than 1), traumatic life events,[4] and parental psychiatric disorders (e.g., suicidality, parental substance use disorder, or other parental psychiatric disorders).[5] The neuroimaging data were used to estimate the trajectories of hippocampal, amygdala, and caudate volume by preschool-age ACEs and school-age maternal support. This revealed interesting interactions between maternal support and ACEs, with some differential effects on specific developmental periods.

The estimated trajectories of hippocampal volume by preschool ACEs and school-age maternal support show that those two factors interact. For

---

[3] Barch, D. Workshop presentation—Early Adversity, Emotional Processing, and the Neural Bases of Psychiatric Illness. Available at http://www.nationalacademies.org/hmd/Activities/Aging/BrainHealthAcrossTheLifeSpanWorkshop/2019-JUN-26.aspx (accessed March 12, 2020).

[4] Traumatic life events included parent arrest; parent hospitalization; crash with motor vehicle, plane, or boat; accidental burning, poisoning, or drowning; attacked by an animal; death of adult loved one; death of sibling or peer; domestic violence; hospitalized, visited emergency department, or had invasive medical procedure; man-made disaster; natural disaster; physical abuse; sexual abuse, sexual assault, or rape; witnessed someone threatened with harm, seriously injured, or killed; physical violence or event causing death or severe harm; or other traumatic life event.

[5] Barch noted that each of those ACEs could have its own independent effect, but they were aggregated in this study.

school-age children with low maternal support (i.e., one standardization below the mean), no particularly strong differential effect of high versus low preschool ACEs was observed. However, participants with mean school-age maternal support have some differentiation, with children with lower preschool ACEs having a steeper increase in hippocampal volume than children with higher preschool ACEs. At one standard deviation above the mean—the strongest school-age maternal support—there is greater differentiation among the effects of preschool ACEs. This is not a buffering pattern, Barch said. In a buffering pattern, high maternal support would see little effect of preschool ACEs—the effect would only be strong for children with low maternal support. Instead, these results suggest that optimal brain health requires both factors to be present: low preschool ACEs as well as strong maternal support that continues at least into school age.

Estimated trajectories of amygdala volume by preschool ACEs and school-age maternal support show a pattern that is somewhat similar. In participants with the lowest maternal support, there was some differentiation among low ACEs versus high ACEs that becomes stronger in participants with greater maternal support. The strongest differentiation was seen in participants with high school-age maternal support. The largest amygdala volumes were associated with low preschool ACEs and high school-age maternal support, suggesting that both factors need to be present to optimize brain development.

Not every brain region shows the same effect, however. Estimated trajectories of caudate volume by preschool ACEs and preschool maternal support show a different pattern. Participants with many ACEs start out with a smaller caudate volume, but regardless of the number of ACEs all participants show a downward decline in caudate volume. That is, differences between low and high ACEs are present from very early on but do not change over time. Independent of that effect, there was a main effect of preschool maternal support showing a similar pattern. That is, participants with low preschool maternal support start low, but do not show a difference in decline compared to participants with high preschool maternal support. This phenomenon is different in the hippocampus and the amygdala, regions in which the effects of ACEs and maternal support interact on the trajectories of volume over time.

## Timing of Mental Health Challenges

Barch turned to the timing with which children develop mental health problems and the relationship that has to brain development. Mental health issues can arise anywhere across the life span—children as young as 3 years of age can have clinical depression and anxiety. Some evidence suggests that earlier onset of mental health issues is associated with especially poor outcomes. Two possible explanations are that (1) the issues occur during key developmental periods or (2) the issues disrupt the child's normative developmental experiences, because early onset of mental health issues is associated with greater chronicity. A child who begins to have mental health problems at a very early age but does not receive treatment has a high likelihood of continuing to have mental health problems. Potentially, this could be a type of experience-dependent learning. Living with depression colors a child's developmental experiences and may change the types of learning experiences they have (Gabard-Durnam and McLaughlin, 2019). However, the timing of the onset of depression may also be interacting with various phases of brain development. Different brain areas, functions, and processes mature at different time points, which may also interact with when a child is experiencing depression.

Barch and colleagues explored these questions using data from the longitudinal study, which included measures of depression from school age to late adolescence.[6] Evidence shows that depression is associated with disruptions in reward processing—in reward anticipation and, in some cases, reward receipt. Barch focused on cue-related brain activity that her team observed by having participants complete a reward anticipation task in the neuroimaging sessions. The overall pattern of brain activity across the entire sample was as expected, with activity in both dorsal and ventral striatum as well as ventral medial prefrontal cortex and visual cortex.

Next, the investigators looked across the entire circuit of brain regions thought to be important for reward processing (including the dorsal and the ventral striatum, and the dorsal and rostral anterior cingulate versus specific brain regions) to see if it was related to a child's current depression versus cumulative level of depression. Then they separated out depression at preschool, school age, and later adolescence to look at differential effects. The only relationship seen with current depression was activity in the nucleus accumbens, where greater depression was associated with reduced activity in that region. Looking at cumulative depression revealed much broader effects—reduction in activity in the circuit as a whole as well as in almost every brain region, with a broader effect related to longer cumulative depression.

Depression during the preschool period shows a broad effect in the caudate, the putamen, and the dorsal and the rostral anterior cingulate, but

[6] Barch, D. Workshop presentation—Early Adversity, Emotional Processing, and the Neural Bases of Psychiatric Illness. Available at http://www.nationalacademies.org/hmd/Activities/Aging/BrainHealthAcrossTheLifeSpanWorkshop/2019-JUN-26.aspx (accessed March 12, 2020).

no effect with the nucleus accumbens. Depression in school-age children shows an effect that is less broad, while adolescent depression was associated with the nucleus accumbens. The same pattern of effects is observed when all three age ranges are included, indicating that these are the differential effects of preschool, school age, and adolescent depression. This suggests that earlier-onset depression is associated with broader effects in the cortical limbic circuit, even when controlling for current depression.

Barch shared a hypothesis related to the different effects of cumulative versus current depression. Current depression severity was associated with hyporeactivity of the ventral striatum to anticipation of reward. If such an association between current depressed mood state and ventral striatal hyporeactivity to reward anticipation is present across development, then repeated experience of depression that starts early in childhood could lead to downstream hyporeactivity of a broader cortico-striatal circuit. An early onset of depression may disrupt this network as the child is developing, with a cascading and broad effect.

## Brain Health and Resilience

Early environmental and emotional experiences relate to brain development in ways that are consistent with both experience-expectant and experience-dependent processes. In addition to considering how to measure brain health or resilience, researchers should consider how to measure the factors that promote brain health and resilience. Figure 7-2 is a simplistic model of how violations of experience-expectant input at specific developmental stages, in conjunction with early-occurring mental health challenges (which are not unrelated), can contribute to disrupted development of limbic and cortical regions. These regions are associated with subsequent poor emotion regulation and stress responsivity, which may contribute to mental health and physical health challenges in adolescence and adulthood.

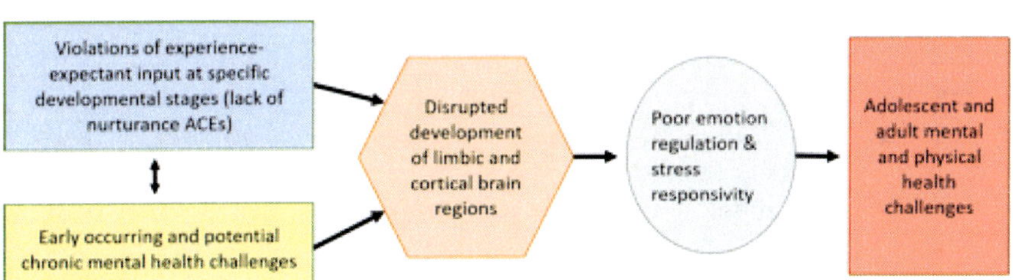


**FIGURE 7-2** Model of disrupted development of limbic and cortical regions.
NOTE: ACE = adverse childhood experience.
SOURCE: As presented by Deanna Barch at the workshop Brain Health Across the Life Span on September 25, 2019.

### Discussion

A participant noted that there appeared to be a negative slope among children with high ACEs as well as high maternal support. Barch agreed that it looks like a negative slope, but it is not a particularly strong effect. The stronger effect is driven by the positive slope of having low ACEs and high maternal support. This was not exactly the pattern Barch's group predicted. They expected to see more of a buffering effect (i.e., very little effect of ACEs with high maternal support); instead, there seems to be more of an additive effect. Another participant asked about potential mechanisms underlying resilience in children with high ACEs who do not receive maternal support, such as self-reliance. Barch replied that she has not looked into this possibility, but she speculated that in children who are removed from a home with a poor maternal relationship, for example, other nurturing caregivers or family members may have an effect on "promoting" resilience.

## THE IMPACT OF EARLY-LIFE STRESS ON NEURODEVELOPMENT

Nim Tottenham, professor in the Department of Psychology at Columbia University, presented on the impact of early-life stress on neurodevelopment. Brain health is age dependent, context dependent, and age appropriate with respect to plasticity and to the tendency or the ability to coordinate with parental cues at age-appropriate times. Humans have a long developmental period for brain development, so it is necessary to pay attention to and support families to improve the brain health of children. Childhood adversity is a leading cause of adult mental health problems, contributing to about one-third of mental illness according to conservative estimates (Kessler et al., 2010). Childhood adversity is one of the major stressors that a developing brain can experience. The large corpus of basic neuroscientific evidence from animal models shows that brain regions such as the amygdala, hippocampus, and prefrontal cortex—which make up the fundamental circuits underlying emotion regulation processes—are highly susceptible to the effects of stress in adulthood and even more so in early life. This is due in part to the rapid growth and potential sensitive periods during this phase of life; it is also due in part to the large extent to which development depends on input from a highly variable outside world (Liston et al., 2006; Magarinos and McEwen, 1995; Mitra et al., 2005; Vyas et al., 2002).

## Influence of Caregivers on Neurodevelopment

Tottenham's presentation explored how input from caregivers in this process affects neurodevelopment. This neurobiology does not develop in isolation; it develops in special species-expected context. Humans spend more time with their parents than other species. In addition to fulfilling basic needs, parents also influence the way a child's brain learns as well as the way the brain constructs itself over time (Tottenham, 2012). Typical children and adolescents have a very robust amygdala response to emotional stimuli early in life. This tends to happen in the absence of the more mature connections among amygdala, prefrontal cortex, and hippocampus that are seen later in adolescence and adulthood. This points to an early period when the nature of the neurobiology may be such that it is highly amenable to influences like individual variations in caregiving (Gabard-Durnam et al., 2014, 2016; Gee et al., 2013b; Silvers et al., 2016; Tottenham and Galván, 2016).

### *Parental Buffering of Aversive Learning in Rats and Humans*

Data from rodent pups show that a parent's regulated presence buffers amygdala activity and aversive learning. During a certain period in postnatal life, the functioning of the amygdala is dependent on the presence or absence of a regulated parent. For example, when the mother rat is in the nest, her presence leads to a neural hormonal cascade that essentially quiets the activity of the pup's amygdala during fear learning. Those processes reverse when the mother is outside of the nest: the same-aged pup's amygdala will now be engaged during fear learning (Moriceau and Sullivan, 2006). That plays out behaviorally in an important way, as demonstrated by placing a peppermint odor that has been paired with a foot shock into one of the arms of a Y maze. If the rat pup acquires that pairing in the absence of its mother, when the amygdala is free to mediate learning, then it avoids the arm that has the odor. However, if the rat pup learns the pairing in the presence of its mother, the mother's presence will block amygdala engagement. This allows competitive learning systems to mediate learning such that fear learning is blocked. These animals tend to show a relative preference for the peppermint odor associated with the mother's presence. This form of learning happens in part because it plays an important role in attachment learning, which must occur during this specific period of life. This suggests that the developmental state of the young altricial brain is designed to coordinate with parental input at certain moments in development.

To investigate whether the type of effect on learning observed in the rats is similarly present humans, a study was conducted with preschool-aged children (Tottenham et al., 2019). The children were presented with a blue square that co-terminated with a terrible noise as well as a triangle that was not paired with any noise. Children learned these pairings either alone or in the physical presence of a parent. Researchers did not observe an effect of the parent's presence during the acquisition phase. After acquisition, the children were placed without their parents into a human Y maze with the triangle on one door and the square on the other in order to look for a behavioral tendency to approach one door over the other.

Children who had been conditioned alone without a parent were more likely than not to avoid the square door, indicating avoidance learning. However, children who had been conditioned in the presence of a parent were more likely than not to show a preference for the square door, which was similar to the behavior seen in the rat pups. This was a within-subjects design, so the same children's learning seemed to be affected by the parent. No effect was seen during acquisition, suggesting that the parent is not simply calming the child, but changing the nature of the learning that occurs. Variability across children is partially explained by cortisol levels, Tottenham added. Children with higher levels of cortisol production were less likely to show this effect of the parent, suggesting some sort of biological constraints on this type of learning.

In a separate study, children were scanned while they looked at pictures of their parents relative to other people's parents. Investigators found that pictures of parents during childhood were effective in dampening the activity of the amygdala (Gee et al., 2014). Although it is not clear whether these are exactly the same processes as shown in rodents, there are some compelling parallels. These types of data suggest that during sensitive periods of childhood, a parent can potentially have large ramifications on the nature of emotion regulation neurobiology that is observed later on in adulthood, reflecting a scaffolding effect. This research provides a foundation for asking questions about what happens to the model when there are severe aberrations in the early caregiving environment.

### Effect of Emotional Neglect or Rejection by Caregiver

Children can experience many types of maltreatment, but Tottenham focused on emotional neglect and/or rejection by the caregiver. Unlike the more obvious signs present in physical neglect or abuse, emotional neglect and rejection effects can be less obvious and often overlooked. This is a pernicious form of maltreatment that is highly comorbid with other forms of maltreatment that children experience. The absence of parental input early in life is not the same as the absence of a threat to the infant. It is a failure to receive needed parent–child intimacy, support, and serve–return dynamic, as well as being a significant stressor during brain development. When considering the role of stress during development, it is important to consider the "stress chronotype" that a child has or experiences—for example, whether the stress experience was limited to the infant period, childhood, adolescence, or whether the stress was chronic (Tottenham and Galván, 2016). Studying different stress chronotypes is valuable because they characterize the experience of many children who are subject to severe adversity. It is important to bear in mind that in many cases, children are still living in those environments at the time of assessment.

*Early Parental Deprivation and Amygdala Responsivity*

Tottenham focused on children who experienced a major early-life stress that was terminated, then followed by a relative absence of stress. In this case, they studied children who experienced early institutional care, which is an extreme form of caregiving neglect or deprivation, and were subsequently adopted into families that provided a very enriched caregiving environment. These children had a significant initial developmental risk followed by a significant rebound in a number of domains after adoption. However, there was significant heterogeneity in their outcomes. At the group level early-life stress is a tremendous risk factor, but there are many individual differences. When children struggle, they are most likely to struggle in the domain broadly defined as emotion regulation, much of which occurs prior to the formation of explicit memory.

Tottenham presented data from children who were placed in institutional care at or near birth and then adopted by their second birthday (Tottenham et al., 2011). They found that previous institutional care is associated with elevated symptoms in the domains of internalizing or externalizing problems in a sample of 373 adolescents, but the data are heterogeneous. To explore what discriminates children at the top of the range from the bottom, they assessed the participants' amygdala responsivity. Previous studies had found evidence of amygdala hyperresponsivity to emotional cues, such as fear faces following early institutional care. These responsivity patterns have been associated with many of the internalizing problems, as well as with behaviors that can be measured in the laboratory. For instance, children with stronger amygdala signals to fear faces were also less likely to make eye contact as measured by eye-tracking measures and as measured by live dyadic interactions (Tottenham et al., 2011).

*Amygdala Hyperactivity Reduces Developmental Plasticity*

Functional connectivity between the amygdala and medial prefrontal cortex reveals age-by-caregiving group interactions. Children with low-risk, no adversity backgrounds were likely to show a more childlike pattern of connectivity between amygdala and prefrontal cortex. Later, in adolescence, a more inhibitory pattern or anticorrelated relationship between the amygdala and prefrontal cortex is typically observed (Gee et al., 2013a). In children with a history of previous institutional care, the connectivity pattern does not look like typically raised children. Instead, it more closely resembles the patterns seen in adolescents and in adults. Tottenham posited that strong amygdala reactivity early in life as a result of stress may actually instantiate earlier formation of these connections with the prefrontal cortex through an activity-based process, leading to a reduction in developmental plasticity (see Figure 7-3). This may represent one means by which early-life stress is reducing neuroplasticity during childhood and adolescence.

It has been posited that these windows of plasticity—or sensitive periods—can be moved by different life experiences (Werker and Hensch, 2015). Caregiving adversity may shift some of these moments of plasticity or truncate them at earlier points within the circuits that have been most affected by early-life adversity (Callaghan and Tottenham, 2016). Tottenham suggested that this may be happening through activity-based processes that have certain immediate benefits to the individual. Evidence suggests that overall, previous institutional care is associated with higher anxiety. However, children in the previous institutional care group show a more adult-like pattern of amygdala-prefrontal connectivity, which

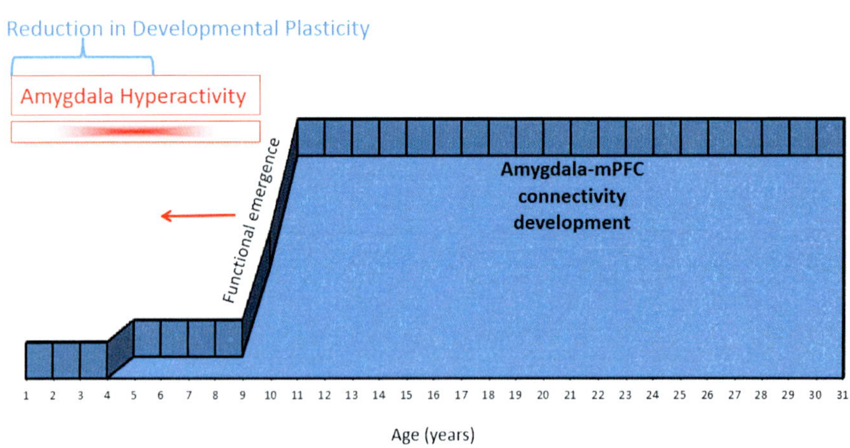


**FIGURE 7-3** Amygdala hyperactivity reduces developmental plasticity.
NOTE: mPFC = medial prefrontal cortex.
SOURCE: As presented by Nim Tottenham at the workshop Brain Health Across the Life Span on September 25, 2019.

indicates lower separation anxiety relative to their peers who did not show that change.

These data suggest that there might be some advantages to emotion regulation processes following early-life stress with this adaptation (Gee et al., 2013a). When the children were followed over 5 years, the children who showed the more adult-like pattern of connectivity were those who were likely to retain the higher anxiety phenotype over time. One hypothesis is that children who showed the more childlike phenotypes through some transactional processes with parents may actually be invoking different caregiving behaviors that could have some benefits on these phenotypes over the long term.

Truncated plasticity also places limits on the developing brain's capacity to respond to parental cues. Unlike the typically raised rat pups that showed the bizarre preference learning in the presence of the parent, animals that had experienced early maltreatment did not show this buffering effect by the parent. Instead, they avoided the negative stimulus. This effect was mediated by the amygdala, such that the presence of the parent was less effective in buffering the amygdala during the fear learning (Moriceau et al., 2009). Similarly, typically raised children showed a decrease in amygdala reactivity to their parents versus strangers that was not seen in children following institutional care. At the group level, this suggests that the parent was less able to modulate the amygdala, but the data show large individual differences; some children might have been showing this amygdala dampening to their parental cues even following very early institutional care.

These individual differences were interrogated longitudinally by splitting the postinstitutional care group into two subgroups: (1) those who showed lowering of the amygdala at time 1, and (2) those who did not, despite having comparable levels of anxiety at initial assessment. Over the 2-year period, those who showed the dampening of the amygdala at time 1 showed the decreases in anxiety over that 2-year period.[7] Those who showed the buffering effects were children who reported higher attachment security. This suggests that even despite the significant adversity, a family can have some powerful effects on shifting this neurobiology.

## Addressing Heterogeneity Among People Exposed to Adversity

Tottenham concluded by noting that early adversity significantly increases the risk for poor mental health, but there is tremendous

[7] Available at http://www.nationalacademies.org/hmd/Activities/Aging/BrainHealthAcrossTheLifeSpanWorkshop/2019-JUN-26.aspx (accessed March 12, 2020).

heterogeneity within groups of people who are exposed to adversity that warrants investigation. Some of these differences might be viewed as potential developmental adaptations, some of which may work for the individuals and others against. The immediate goal is to better understand independent variables in studies of early-life stress, while also considering how environmental needs develop and change with age. This heterogeneity is present within subgroupings of people who experienced early adversity, such as people who experienced domestic foster care and people who experienced international adoption with institutional care. This indicates that there may be specific experiences that transcend these traditional recruitment boundaries.

Her group's current approach is to invite children who have experienced various types of caregiving experiences—both positive experiences and adversities—and, through data-driven processes, to cluster those children either on their brain behavior phenotypes or on their caregiving experiences. These clusters can also include adversities that are not related to caregiving per se. Preliminary data are beginning to reveal some evidence of meaningful clusters, although there is still heterogeneity within the clusters and there are some factors that transcend these different boundaries.

## INTEGRATING COMPLEX AND PERSONALIZED DATA TO UNDERSTAND NORMAL AND ABNORMAL BRAIN NETWORK DEVELOPMENT

Satterthwaite described two studies that integrate complex and personalized measures of network development throughout youth and adolescence with a focus on brain health. He explained that the rationale for studying brain development is increasingly clear. Convergent lines of evidence from animal models, human epidemiological studies, and translational studies suggest that most major neuropsychiatric conditions can be conceptualized as disorders of development. This domain of research seeks to understand how the brain develops normally and then to understand how abnormal patterns of brain development are associated with different forms of psychopathology.

The ultimate goal of describing major mental illness in terms of abnormal trajectories of brain development is to allow for earlier diagnosis and intervention with more effective treatments in order to achieve improved functional outcomes for people living with these conditions. This work requires large-scale data that allow for sampling across multiple age ranges in both healthy and affected children. In his presentation, Satterthwaite presented neuroimaging data from a complex large-scale initiative called the Philadelphia Neurodevelopmental Cohort (PNC), which focuses on characterizing brain and behavior interaction with genetics. The cohort included 1,600 children aged 8–22 years, with a balanced mix of males and females and of Caucasians and African Americans that reflects the local Philadelphia population (Satterthwaite et al., 2014).

## Network Modularity as a Key Measure of Brain Health

Satterthwaite used selection neuroimaging data from the PNC to focus on structural and functional brain networks. Unlike neurological conditions in which there is a clear lesion and focality, psychiatric conditions are increasingly conceptualized as connectopathies—that is, disorders of how the brain communicates. Brain networks can be measured both structurally and functionally. Structural brain networks can be reconstructed with diffusion imaging tractography techniques, while functional brain networks can be estimated with functional magnetic resonance imaging (fMRI).

Network modularity is a key feature of brain development as well as aging. Although measures of brain health are not yet sufficiently refined to be clinically actionable, available data suggest that network modularity is a key measure (Satterthwaite et al., 2014). A network module is a collection of brain regions that are tightly connected to each other and weakly connected to other parts of the brain. These correspond to functional subsystems of the brain, as defined by conversion evidence from task fMRI, lesion studies, and animal studies. This modularity can be visualized using spring-embedded rendering to depict how the tightly connected brain regions are brought together and the weakly connected brain regions are pushed apart, highlighting the network modules.

One of the most widely replicated findings in developmental cognitive neuroscience is that this modularity evolves dramatically throughout childhood and adolescence (Fair et al., 2007). Intramodular connections are much more likely to strengthen than weaken with age, which causes modules to become more defined during adolescence (Satterthwaite et al., 2014). Satterthwaite's group recently showed that structural brain networks undergo a similar process of modular segregation—modules become refined and prominent, with more connectivity within a module and less connectivity between modules. These modules are present but are relatively indistinct in younger children, but they become much more defined as the children grow up. This modular segregation has functional consequences. The development of executive function during this period is mediated by the degree to which this network topology develops in the brain, with modules shifting toward more specialized functions (Baum et al., 2017). However, this type of analysis only looks at simple, low-dimensional summary measures of network structure and only at executive function, which is just a single domain of cognition. A more clinically relevant approach would be to look across all clinical domains in psychiatry and simultaneously map these to abnormalities in the high-dimensional topology of the connectome.

## Data Integration to Understand Abnormal Network Development

Satterthwaite described a recent study that used machine-learning techniques to integrate complex clinical data with high-dimensional imaging data. First, he described how the approach used in this project is a departure from the case-control design of clinical studies (e.g., comparing a person with a diagnosis of depression to a healthy person), which does not address two central challenges in integrative psychiatric neuroscience. The conceptual challenge is that clinical diagnostic categories as codified in clinical practice are not clean biological classes, owing to vast heterogeneity and the frequency of comorbidities. In other words, they do not carve nature at the joints in a clear way. For example, depression is a large category that is unlikely to represent a single biological phenomenon, given the amount of heterogeneity that has been demonstrated and the number of comorbidities that occur with the condition, such as anxiety.

### *Dimensionality*

The methodological challenge is that the data are highly dimensional. Typical case-control designs that ignore heterogeneity and comorbidity are often very hypothesis driven, thus they miss the opportunity to collect other rich data. Instead, this project takes a discovery science approach using machine learning to define data-driven links between functional brain networks and psychiatric symptoms. He said that in essence, this "lets the brain teach us what the dimensions should be." He explained that typical functional networks use atlases with hundreds of nodes that cover the entire brain; when this is taken to a connectivity matrix, connections between each of these nodes can create a common network with tens of thousands of edges (Xia et al., 2018). This is relatively high-dimensional data.

A problem that is just as substantial, but even more commonly ignored, is that clinical data also have reasonable dimensionality. Standardized psychiatric interviews include hundreds of questions about symptoms, but most psychiatric imaging studies take a very reduced look at these data—for example, by looking only at amygdala connectivity and the rest of the brain, instead of looking at the entire connectivity matrix. Similarly, a clinical case-control study of depression would typically ignore other symptoms and collapse the depression items into a single categorical diagnosis.

A common alternative is to try to integrate the data through data reduction, for instance, by looking parsimoniously at a small number of brain networks instead of looking at all 35,000 connections or by summarizing itemwise clinical data into a four- or five-factor model. Although this approach is reasonable, it is based on the assumption—which is not well supported by evidence—that the biological scale of the abnormalities matches with the scale of data reduction. Another alternative is to try to directly integrate high-dimensional brain data with available granular clinical data using sparse canonical correlation analysis (sCCA).[8]

## Identifying Linked Dimensions of Psychopathology and Functional Connectivity

The approach taken in the study Satterthwaite presented uses sCCA to build a linear combination of brain features that predict a linear combination of clinical features in a data-driven manner (Xia et al., 2018). Through a process of permutation testing and correction for multiple comparisons, sCCA can be used to identify linked dimensions of psychopathology and functional connectivity. In this case, the study identified the dimensions of mood, psychosis, fear, and externalizing behavior. A first step in looking at the data was to plot the brain connectivity score versus the clinical dimension score, which revealed tight relationships between the brain and the clinical dimension and allowed for identifying the most highly rated clinical item in each of the dimensions. For example, the most highly rated item in the mood dimension is "feeling sad" (Xia et al., 2018). Boot-strap resampling anyalysis was used to understand which clinical items significantly contribute to each dimension. Figure 7-4 is a ring plot that is laid out with classic discrete clinical diagnoses in the outer ring. In the inner rings are the loadings of the clinical items in each dimension.

Investigators found that the clinical item loadings accord with clinical experience, but they also cross diagnostic boundaries (Xia et al., 2018). These data-driven dimensions of psychopathology generally cohere with the clinical diagnostic categories to a great extent, but they also bleed across them in a graded way. The psychosis dimension has significant loadings in the mania items, for instance, which makes sense given the

[8] sCCA is an updated version of an older statistical technique called canonical correlation analysis, which is limited by the requirement to have more samples than features in the model. sCCA imposes sparsity constraints that allow the model to have more features than samples.

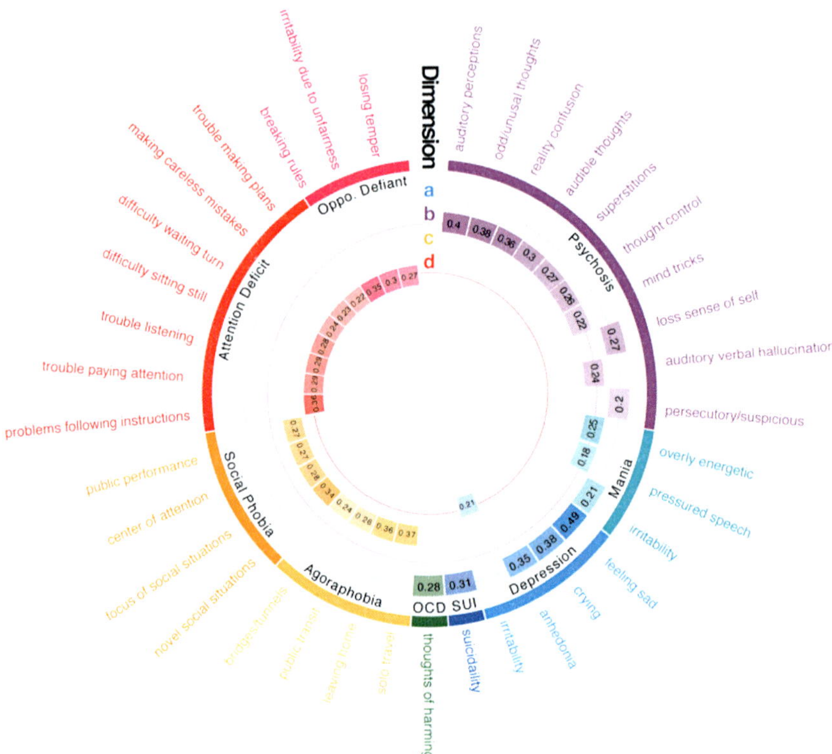


**FIGURE 7-4** Clinical item loadings accord with clinical experience and cross diagnostic boundaries.
NOTE: OCD = obsessive–compulsive disorder; OPPO = oppositional; SUI = suicidality.
SOURCES: As presented by Ted Satterthwaite at the workshop Brain Health Across the Life Span on September 25, 2019; Xia et al., 2018.

genetic overlap between bipolar disorder and psychotic disorders. Furthermore, Satterthwaite and colleagues found that specific differences of functional connectivity define each dimension, but there are key features that are present across each dimension, such as a loss of modular segregation.

Studies of typical brain development show that modular segregation evolves throughout childhood and adolescence and supports executive function. In these data-driven dimensions of psychopathology, each of these dimensions is associated with a loss of this normative modular segregation (Xia et al., 2018). A replication sample generated largely convergent results with the initial discovery sample, although the psychosis dimension was not replicated. Together, this indicates that data-driven dimensions of psychopathology can link abnormalities and functional connectivity. Modular segregation is a common feature across the dimensions, suggesting that it is an important aspect of brain health as the brain develops (Xia et al., 2018).

## Personalized Development of Network Topography

The second study presented by Satterthwaite was designed to work toward personalizing measures of functional connectivity. Typically, all the brain images from participants in a study are registered to a standard group atlas, with an implicit assumption that networks are in the same anatomical location for each person. Satterthwaite's study addresses a major limitation of the first study he presented as well as most studies of functional brain networks conducted until recently: the idea that the functional networks in the brain are laid out similarly across individuals.

### *Functional Topography Varies Across Individuals*

However, recent evidence from multiple groups has shown that this assumption is demonstrably false. For example, work using the Midnight Scan Club[9] dataset shows remarkable heterogeneity in the spatial layout of these functional networks on the anatomic cortex, which has been replicated in multiple datasets using independent methods (Bijsterbosch et al., 2018; Gordon et al., 2017; Kong et al., 2019; Li et al., 2017). Furthermore, these studies reveal the heterogeneity in functional topography, or the spatial layout of these functional networks, varies by location in the brain. Functional topography varies most across individuals in the higher-order association cortex, which are the regions of the brain most relevant in psychiatric illness. Across different sets, the most variability is present in the frontoparietal control network and in the ventral attention network. However, it is not yet understood how this individualized functional topography evolves in development or how it associates with important domains of healthy behavior, such as executive function.

Nonnegative matrix factorization is a machine-learning technique that can be used for identifying brain networks in individuals (Li et al., 2018), and it allows for defining 17 networks per person on a subject-specific basis (Cui et al., 2020). Single-subject data show that the spatial layout of these networks varies between individuals. For example, looking into frontoparietal networks and the ventral attention networks either on a continuously loaded basis or on a binary basis shows that they vary

[9] See the Midnight Scan Club dataset at https://www.openfmri.org/dataset/ds000224 (accessed November 13, 2019).

in terms of their placement on the anatomic cortex (Cui et al., 2020). The networks with the highest variability are in the frontoparietal control network and the ventral attention system, which are key networks for executive function (Cui et al., 2020).

To explore how these highly variable networks evolve throughout the adolescent period, which is a critical period for the development of brain health and the period in which many neuropsychiatric symptoms begin to emerge, Cui and colleagues created a total network representation. This is a simple measure of each of the individualized networks that summarizes how much space on an individual cortex each functional network occupies. They found that total network representation did not associate with age (which was surprising), but it was strongly associated with executive function (Cui et al., 2020). Children and adolescents who perform better in executive tasks have more total network representation allotted to systems that are important for executive function, like the frontoparietal control network and the ventral attention network.

To move beyond the simple summary measure to the overall multivariate pattern of how the functional topography is laid out in the brain, researchers used split-half data and machine-learning techniques to predict executive function in completely unseen data with a relatively high degree of accuracy (Cui et al., 2020). The most important weights were seen in the ventral attention system and in the frontoparietal control network, suggesting that the individualized layout of functional network topography could be a very important measure of brain health in adolescents. Finally, they looked at whether the overall complex pattern of functional topography was associated with age. Even though the summary measure of the total network representation did not seem to change with age, it was possible to predict age from the functional network topography even more accurately than executive function could be predicted. In fact, it was refinement within association networks that predicted age. The total size of these networks did not change over the age span, but the borders of the network were sharpened. This suggests that these networks are differentiating throughout the developmental period, in a process reminiscent of the network-wide segregation process. Satterthwaite added that these highly variable brain networks, with functional topography that varies across individuals, have certain fundamental properties of cortical organization.

Variability in the frontoparietal control network and the ventral attention system align with a high degree of evolutionary expansion, low cortical myelin content, and high cerebral blood flow (Cui et al., 2020). This is consistent with an account whereby association networks evolve and become untethered from rigid developmental programs. This process is probably beneficial in many ways, because it allows for interindividual variability and adaptability as children are developing. However, it also comes at a metabolic cost and could potentially lead to higher vulnerability to neuropsychiatric syndromes during the critical period of adolescence.

## BRAIN NETWORK AGING AND HEALTH ACROSS THE ADULT LIFE SPAN

Gagan Wig, associate professor of behavioral and brain sciences at the Center for Vital Longevity at the University of Texas at Dallas, presented on brain network aging and health across the adult life span, with a focus on novel measures of brain health. Even in the absence of disease, aging is associated with progressive changes in cognition (Park and Reuter-Lorenz, 2009). However, simply comparing endpoints between younger and older adults is inadequate to understanding cognitive health decline. Aging also varies widely across individuals, with longitudinal data demonstrating how perceptual speed declines within an individual over age at very different rates (Wilson et al., 2002). Although variance can be helpful in understanding how steeper declines might be related to degenerative processes versus typical aging, understanding the parameter space of healthy aging requires inquiry into the brain associates that accompany those behavioral observations.

Multiple imaging-based measures of the brain can be used to characterize aging, including functional activation (Cabeza et al., 1997), structure of gray matter (Raz et al., 1997) and white matter (O'Sullivan et al., 2001), metabolism (Oh et al., 2016), and dopamine binding. However, none of these measures is considered a standard measure of brain health, because it is not yet well understood how the information that is embedded in the signals provided by these tests correspond to individual variation in brain health and potential health outcomes.

Wig suggested that understanding brain health and risk of decline will require examining multiple brain measures together as well as identifying novel measures. His group conducts work based on the hypothesis that resting-state brain network organization is an important biomarker (for lack of a better term) of age-related cognitive decline. The network approach may be the most appropriate framework that is currently available for understanding cognition. Analyzing resting-state networks involves four main steps: identifying parcellated nodes of the brain, extracting the time course for every node and computing pairwise correlations, building node-to-node correlation matrices for each subject, and then graphing a theoretic analysis of network structure (Bullmore and Sporns, 2009; Wig et al., 2011). The work he described focuses on the graph structure in terms of aging.

## Desirable Features of Measures of Health in Aging Brains

To provide context for thinking about measures of brain health, Wig outlined a set of desirable features for measures of brain health as people age: ease of collection, reliability, validity, and changeability. Validity of brain health measures can be characterized in different ways, such as having continuous variation across the adult life span and not just at the endpoints or being related to cognition, even in "typical" ranges. It could also be described as being moderated by measures related to general health, environment, and lifestyle or by its predictive value in warning of impending dysfunction or adverse event. Changeability is desirable because it can be modified in an ideal situation.

## Differences in Brain Network Organization Across the Adult Life Span

Evidence is emerging that resting-state brain networks in young adults are organized into communities—described by Satterthwaite in terms of modularity—that correspond to functionally distinct brain systems (Power et al., 2011). Wig's group is applying that observation in the context of healthy aging and how that organization differs across the adult life span. They are using the Dallas Lifespan Brain Study dataset, which includes data from more than 300 subjects sampled across a broad segment of the adult life span collected via T1, DTI, and BOLD functional scans (multiple tasks and rest). Starting with the rest data, Wig's group has worked to minimize known sources of variance by minimizing the influence of movement and ensuring quality control of the T1 and BOLD data, which are both susceptible to movement-related artifacts (Power et al., 2014; Savalia et al., 2017).

The topography of large-scale functional brain systems is largely consistent across the healthy adult life span, indicating that healthy aging is not accompanied by a massive reconfiguration of basic modular structure (Han et al., 2018).[10] Inherent in this description of functional systems is the idea that modularity requires dense within-system connections and sparser between-system connections (Power et al., 2011). Although this concept may underpin functional specialization of a network, the segregation of network communities can change over time.

[10] To avoid the limitation of fixed node atlases in network descriptions (described by Satterthwaite) they create parcellations at every age cohort level.

### *Effect of Aging on Network Segregation*

Having network communities that are segregated, but still able to communicate with one another, requires a fine balance of connections both within and between the communities. This confers functional specialization as well as some interaction between them (Wig, 2017). As functionally specialized communities in the network become more segregated, they become increasingly disconnected; if they become less segregated, they run the risk of becoming undifferentiated.

Wig's group hypothesized that functionally specialized networks in healthy young adults would be situated roughly in the middle of this spectrum. To explore whether aging has an effect on this basic property, they took the nodes as a function of the system and classified them according to whether the connections were within or between systems and used the weighted average of the various connection types as the measure of segregation. They found that older age was associated with decreased segregation of large-scale brain systems. With increasing age, the connectivity within the functional systems decreases but the connectivity between systems increases (Chan et al., 2014).

Figure 7-5 is a spring-bedding diagram showing that increasingly sparser connectivity is associated with increasing age fanning outward (i.e., in the blue system, which corresponds to the visual system). The interactions between the association systems (i.e., within the circle in purple, yellow, and green, corresponding to the cingulo-opercular control system, frontal-parietal control system, and dorsal attention system, respectively) tend to increase, leading to the observation of decreasing segregation.

### *Reliability of the Relationship Between Brain System Segregation and Adult Age*

With respect to reliability of the relationship between system segregation and adult age, the age-versus-system segregation relationship has now been observed across multiple studies using different methods (Betzel et al., 2014; Cassady et al., 2019; Chong et al., 2019; Geerligs et al., 2014; Grady et al., 2016; Han et al., 2018; King et al., 2017; Shaw et al., 2015; Song et al., 2014; Spreng et al., 2016; Zonneveld et al., 2019). Wig's laboratory has also carried out independent replications based on other data sets that support the relationship between the system segregation measure and age. Additionally, his group has looked at whether system segregation is a reliable measure of an individual's brain network organization by using resting-state data from young adults collected on two different days, finding the measure to be strong enough that there is reason to believe it might be a useful way of thinking about individual-level network organization.

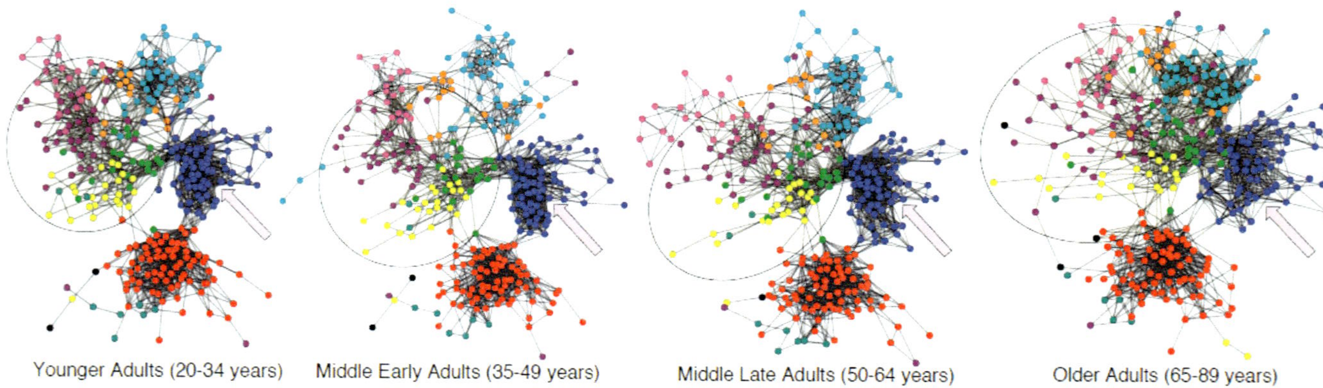


**FIGURE 7-5** Effect of aging on network segregation.
SOURCES: As presented by Gagan Wig at the workshop Brain Health Across the Life Span on September 25, 2019; Chan et al., 2014.

*Relationship Between Brain System Segregation and Cognitive Ability*

Features of the Dallas Lifespan Brain Study dataset were also helpful for exploring how measures of the brain relate to cognitive ability. The data show that increasing segregation is related to long-term memory (Chan et al., 2014). When the age effect is accounted for, people that have more segregated systems have better memory ability independent of age (Chan et al., 2014). In other words, some older adults with very high system segregation have relatively higher memory scores, while some younger adults with lower system segregation have poorer memory scores (Chan et al., 2014). The trajectory of these individuals over time is a research direction of interest.

## Modifiers of System Segregation Across the Adult Life Span

Wig's group has also looked for other modifiers of system segregation across the adult life span, such as the role of the individual's environment, by using a bigger sample from the Dallas Lifespan Brain Study (Chan et al., 2018).[11] In adults, lower socioeconomic status (SES) is associated with worse cognition (Koster et al., 2005) and greater risk of Alzheimer's disease (Stern et al., 1994), so Wig's group explored whether SES relates to this measure of brain organization. SES is a crude construct, but it does give a sense of access to resources, nutrition, health care, cognitive stimulation, and levels of stress.

In this case, Wig's group defined SES by education and occupational status. The analysis, using continuous measures of age and SES, found that lower SES was associated with reduced system segregation in middle-age adulthood, but not in younger or older adults (see Figure 7-6). The relationship persists when controlling for demographics, physical health, mental health, cognitive ability, and a measure of childhood SES based on parental education. Because the measure does not differ for older adults, Wig suggested that this indicates a survivor bias in lower SES older adults (Chan et al., 2018). For younger adults, he suggested that the commonly used SES measure is inappropriate, because they may have evolving educational and occupational states.

[11] A second round of data collection was conducted with relaxed exclusion criteria to include people with lower education and chronic health conditions, providing a more population-representative sample.

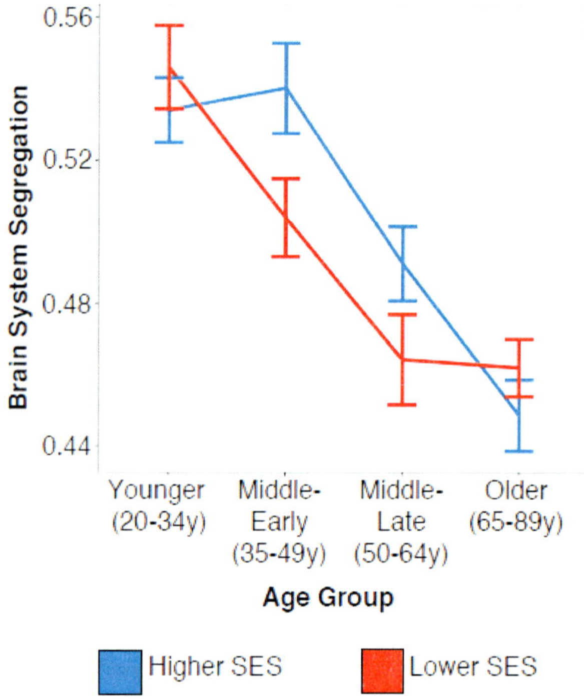


**FIGURE 7-6** Lower socioeconomic status (SES) is associated with reduced system segregation in middle-age adulthood.
NOTES: Participants: Dallas Lifespan Brain Study (DLBS); N = 359; SES defined by education and occupational status.
SOURCES: As presented by Gagan Wig at the workshop Brain Health Across the Life Span on September 25, 2019; Chan et al., 2018.

### Future Research Directions

Wig concluded by outlining a set of his group's future research directions. Rather than looking at cross-sectional data, his group is focused on examining networks within an individual by bringing together multiple large longitudinal datasets to explore whether brain networks change as an individual grows older in both health and disease, whether brain network organization is modified by changes in brain degeneration, and if brain network patterns can be used to predict who may be vulnerable to brain disorders. The group is also looking at which aspects of an individual's environment mediate the SES–brain network relationships in a study focused on community-based, middle-age adults who are at or near the household poverty line. Through longitudinal assessment of changes in brain network organization and cognition, Wig's group plans to extensively characterize changes in health and lifestyle over time using biological measures, survey-based measures, and other techniques. Work focused on interventions is also under way to explore whether the system segregation of an individual's brain network can be changed.

One of the studies involves engaged learning of new skills by older adults, based on the idea that maintaining brain health and cognition involves continuous learning. Another study is looking at the potential for precision brain stimulation to alter network organization. Participants are receiving extensive transcranial magnetic stimulation at specific parcels (brain regions) based on the individual's specific brain topography to determine whether there is a change in network segregation as a function of stimulation location.

## PANEL DISCUSSION ON THE WAY FORWARD IN MEASUREMENT AND RESEARCH

Damien Fair, associate professor of behavioral neuroscience, associate professor of psychiatry, and associate scientist at the Advanced Imaging Research Center at the Oregon Health & Science University, asked the panelists to comment on the types of research needed to make the leap from the conceptual to the actionable in long-term brain health.

### Brain Health Growth Charts

Barch highlighted a challenge in measuring the development and decline of brain health throughout the life span. It is possible to observe group differences and identify individuals, but it is not yet possible to determine which people need extra clinical intervention. This will require developing the appropriate psychometrics, measurement tools, databases, and study designs. She suggested tracking brain health through a "growth chart" to capture individual changes over time, as is already done for physical growth measurements. Tottenham remarked that creating brain health growth charts would be very useful, but a potential complication is the need to integrate context-specific environmental factors into the system.

Behavioral outcomes have an additional layer of complexity in that whether or not certain outcomes are healthy is contextualized by the specific environment. Manly noted that physical growth charts assume universality and variance in their predictions of important outcomes; they are generally intended to be screening tools rather than diagnostic tools. Brain health growth charts have the potential to be used as a screening tool for inappropriate purposes that might actually widen disparities rather than narrowing them, Manly cautioned. A participant added that body type and physiological factors such as insulin resistance can substantially affect brain development, so brain–body interactions would be important to capture.

### Leveraging Electronic Health Records Systems

Health systems that have integrated electronic health record systems are at an advantage in this regard, said Satterthwaite. Such systems are already capturing important biologically based measures that could be easily scaled—through mobile platforms or otherwise—and then linked to meaningful health outcomes. Currently, differential treatment response to measures of brain health is a major gap in the literature that will need to be addressed to make this research clinically actionable. Building systems of informatics could also help to link biological measures to health outcomes. Fair highlighted this suggestion as a potentially actionable item that could have a relatively large effect.

### Identifying Practical Measures with Clinical Usefulness

Lis Nielsen, chief of the individual behavioral processes branch of the Division of Behavioral and Social Research at the National Institute on Aging, commented about the work on network differentiations and patterns over development. Currently, these kinds of measures cannot feasibly be captured on a broad scale for use as diagnostic or screening tools. She was interested in how mapping network development over time relates to the evolution of the entire range of functions that those networks represent. Mapping those functions onto simple cognitive assessments, in order to capture measures in larger populations or in clinics, could potentially shed light on the drivers of network differentiation or interaction that enable the network functions.

Nielsen asked what research would be needed to facilitate the ability to capture this simply by assessing cognition and other functions. Wig replied that network functions correspond to systems of the brain that are functionally distinct. Data show that increasing differences among measures are associated with changes in activity of the specific regions that tie the networks together. His group is conducting a newer study that includes multiple features to identify relationships to other measures that could feasibly be collected on a larger scale. It is not practical to collect neuroimaging data from everyone, so the aim is to identify measures or sets of features that relate to and mediate the relationships observed in imaging studies, but which can be collected simply and quickly for use in health care settings.

### Balancing Conceptual Research with Practical Interventions

Barch commented that the focus on individual differences in brain health that are unrelated to environmental factors may distract from efforts to address brain health issues that are known consequences of well-established factors—such as early adversity, SES, poverty, and stress—that also influence physical health (e.g., insulin resistance). Research on the biological bases of brain development and developing measures of brain health outcomes would be helpful in many ways, but there will always be individual variation, and this work should not preclude efforts to intervene on environmental factors that are known to influence brain development. For example, relatively simple interventions, such as a modest income transfer to families living with housing or nutritional instability, would likely have positive effects on the brain health as well as physical health of children in those families. She emphasized that the focus on measuring outcomes and identifying people with brain health issues should not come at the expense of implementing strategies to address the environmental factors that are driving those brain issues.

Tottenham agreed, noting that measures such as insulin resistance are actually outcome measures of a number of different factors. While it may theoretically be easier to change external environmental factors than genetic influences, for example, these types of interventions are constrained by a range of political, economic, and social forces on a practical level. She reiterated that at the very least, 30 percent of mental illness is attributable to childhood adversities. These childhood adversity factors are entirely modifiable, but doing so requires a society to collectively decide to improve them.

### Geographic Diversity in Brain Health

A participant noted that because brain health outcomes have wide geographic diversity, research should seek to better understand the mechanisms that underlie this diversity and how factors such as place of birth versus place of current residence interact with each other and predict outcomes. Barch noted that much of that geographic diversity reflects variation in different facets of SES, such as quality of schools, median income, and other metrics. Urbanicity also has both positive and negative effects on mental health outcomes that depend on factors such as minority status. She added that there is a dearth of neuroimaging data from rural areas, so it is unclear if the same types of relationships hold as in urban areas.

## Next Steps

Fair suggested focusing on next steps in identifying interventions that would have the most "bang for the buck." For instance, delaying school start times to allow adolescents to get a little more sleep is a relatively small change that would have a great effect.

### *Guidelines for Improving Brain Health*

Stephanie Cacioppo, director of the brain dynamics laboratory, assistant professor of psychiatry and behavioral neuroscience, and assistant professor at the Grossman Institute for Neuroscience at the University of Chicago Pritzker School of Medicine, suggested developing specific, practical guidelines for improving brain health that would be analogous to existing guidelines on how to improve physical health. Barch commented that there is a range of commonsense good practices that can improve brain health, such as exercise and sleep. However, she warned against framing that kind of information to imply incorrectly that it will prevent the occurrence of Alzheimer's disease or other brain disorders with underlying genetic factors.

Tottenham suggested adding Maslow's hierarchy of needs to the list of good practices for brain health, but that these needs should be developmentally tailored. Notably, for infants and young children, availability of a reliable caregiver should be added to the list of other survival needs like food, water, and shelter at the most fundamental level of the hierarchy. Adequate, stable caregiving would be a basic need early on, but it is not necessarily a fundamental basic survival need for an older individual.

### *Clinical Assessment of Environmental Factors*

Nielsen suggested that importing the assessment of environmental variables into the clinical context may be low-hanging fruit. There is evidence that individuals with a history of early life adversity may be differentially responsive to treatments for depression and other mental disorders, but clinics do not typically ask about those factors. There may be value in collecting such data to examine implications for preventive and treatment interventions addressing a range of cognitive and emotional disorders. Clinical assessment of personality, which can predict a portion of a person's risk for Alzheimer's disease, could also be useful in informing treatment decisions, and awareness of risk could potentially encourage people to mitigate other risk factors for the disease. Similarly, evidence about differential response to depression treatment as a function of early-life adversity could inform interventions and treatment decisions in a way that does not require any kind of new brain measure.

# Appendix A

# Speaker Biographical Sketches

**Huda Akil, Ph.D.,** is focused on understanding the neurobiology of emotions, including pain, anxiety, depression, and substance abuse. Research in the Akil laboratory is focused on understanding the neurobiology of emotions, including pain, anxiety, depression, and substance abuse. Early on, Dr. Akil's research focused on the role of the endorphins and their receptors in pain and stress responsiveness. She provided the first physiological evidence for a role of endogenous opioids in the brain and showed that endorphins are activated by stress and cause pain inhibition, a phenomenon termed *stress-induced analgesia*. Dr. Akil defined how the posttranslational processing of opioid precursors is modulated by stress, and demonstrated the coordinated actions of the neuropeptide products on behavior. Dr. Akil collaborated with Dr. Stanley Watson in a series of studies characterizing the anatomy of the opioid peptides and their receptors. The Akil and Watson research groups collaboratively cloned two types of opioid receptors and conducted structure–function analyses defining the molecular basis of high affinity and selectivity toward the endogenous ligands. Dr. Akil is a member of the National Academy of Sciences and the National Academy of Medicine.

**B. J. Casey, Ph.D.,** is a professor of psychology at Yale University and an adjunct professor at the Weill Cornell Medical College in New York City, where she holds appointments in the Departments of Psychiatry and Neuroscience and an adjunct appointment at The Rockefeller University. Dr. Casey is a world leader in human neuroimaging and its use in typical and atypical development. She skillfully uses brain imaging to uniquely examine developmental transitions across the life span, especially during the period of adolescence. Her work is grounded in translational studies from genetically altered mice to humans to patients, developing models for several mental heath problems that affect millions of young people today. Her studies have begun to inform when and how to target treatments to the individual based on age and genetic profile (i.e., precision medicine) and her discoveries have been highlighted by NPR, PBS, *The New York Times*, *The Wall Street Journal*, and *National Geographic* and have implications for juvenile justice and mental health policy reform. Dr. Casey has served on several advisory boards, including the National Institute of Mental Health (NIMH) Board of Scientific Counselors and NIMH Council; the Scientific Advisory Board for NARSAD; the Advisory Board for the Human Connectome Project—Life Span Study; the National Academies of Sciences, Engineering, and Medicine's Board of Children, Youth, and Families; and the National Academies committees on the science of adolescent risk taking, assessing juvenile justice reform, and sports-related concussions in youth. She has received funding from NIMH, the National Institute on Drug Abuse, the National Institute of Child Health and Human Development, the National Science Foundation, the John Merck Fund, the Dana Foundation, and the MacArthur Foundation. She has been asked to present her work on the adolescent brain to congressional staff on Capitol Hill, to the Washington State Supreme Court, and to federal judges around the country. She is the recipient of numerous awards, including an honorary doctorate from Utrecht University in the Netherlands, and she is the author of nearly 200 publications. Dr. Casey is someone who takes the training of the next generation of scientists as seriously as her own research, about which she is passionate.

**Damien A. Fair, P.A.-C., Ph.D.,** is an associate professor of behavioral neuroscience and psychiatry at the Oregon Health & Science University (OHSU), as well as an associate scientist at OHSU's Advanced Imaging Research Center, principal investigator (PI) and co-PI on studies of typical and atypical brain development and attention-deficit hyperactivity disorder (ADHD) brain development. His laboratory focuses on mechanisms and principles that underlie the developing brain. The majority of this work uses functional magnetic resonance imaging (fMRI) and resting state functional connectivity MRI to assess typical and atypical populations. A second focus has become testing the feasibility of using various functional and structural MRI techniques in translational studies of developmental neuropsychiatric disorders (e.g., ADHD and autism). Dr. Fair's lab is exploring ways to better characterize individual patients with these psychopathologies to help guide future diagnostic, therapeutic, and genetic studies.

**Jennifer J. Manly, Ph.D.,** is a professor of neuropsychology in neurology at the Gertrude H. Sergievsky Center and the Taub Institute for Research in Aging and Alzheimer's disease at Columbia University. She completed her graduate training in neuropsychology at the San Diego State University/University of California, San Diego, Joint Doctoral Program in clinical psychology. After a clinical internship at Brown University, she completed a postdoctoral fellowship at Columbia University. Her research on cultural, medical, and genetic predictors of cognitive aging and Alzheimer's disease among African Americans and Hispanics has been funded by the National Institute on Aging and the Alzheimer's Association. She has authored more than 100 peer-reviewed publications and 8 chapters. In 2002 she was awarded the Early Career Award from Division 40 of the American Psychological Association (APA), and in 2004 she was elected a fellow of APA. She serves on the Department of Health and Human Services' Advisory Council on Alzheimer's Research, Care, and Services, and she is a member of the Alzheimer's Association Medical & Scientific Research Board. She currently serves as a member at large on the Board of Governors of the International Neuropsychological Society.

**Bruce S. McEwen, Ph.D.,** was the Alfred E. Mirsky Professor at The Rockefeller University. A major figure in behavioral neuroendocrinology, Dr. McEwen produced a massive body of important work on the roles of steroid hormones in reproductive behavior, brain development, gene expression in the brain, brain plasticity in adulthood, and the effects of stress on age-related brain degeneration that causes cognitive deficits. As a neuroscientist and a neuroendocrinologist, he studied environmentally regulated, variable gene expression in the brain mediated by circulating steroid hormones and endogenous neurotransmitters in relation to brain sexual differentiation and the actions of sex, stress, and thyroid hormones on the adult brain. He combined molecular, anatomical, pharmacological, physiological, and behavioral methodologies and related his findings to human clinical information. He found receptors for adrenal steroids in the hippocampus that are transcription factors, a discovery that triggered an ever-growing number of studies throughout the world on the neural effects of adrenal steroids and stress on the hippocampus. Dr. McEwen was a member of the National Academy of Sciences and the National Academy of Medicine.

**Bruce L. Miller, M.D.,** holds the A.W. and Mary Margaret Clausen Distinguished Professorship in Neurology at the University of California,

San Francisco (UCSF). He directs the busy UCSF dementia center where patients in the San Francisco Bay Area and beyond receive comprehensive clinical evaluations. His goal is the delivery of model care to all of the patients who enter the clinical and research programs at the UCSF Memory and Aging Center. Dr. Miller is a behavioral neurologist focused on dementia with special interests in brain and behavior relationships as well as the genetic and molecular underpinnings of disease. Dr. Miller is a member of the National Academy of Medicine.

# Appendix B

# Workshop Agenda

Brain Health Across the Life Span: A Workshop
September 24–25, 2019
2101 Constitution Avenue, NW
Washington, DC

**Workshop Objectives**

1. What are accepted definitions of *brain health* and *resilience*?
2. What are the key elements to measure status of *brain health* and its *resilience* across the life span?
3. What additional research questions can be addressed to increase our understanding of brain plasticity throughout the life span?

**TUESDAY, SEPTEMBER 24, 2019**

**Room 120**

| | |
|---|---|
| 9:30–10:00 am | **Welcome and Opening Remarks**<br>Richard D. Olson<br>Director, Division of Prevention Science<br>Office of Disease Prevention and Health Promotion<br>Office of the Assistant Secretary for Health<br>Department of Health and Human Services |

Admiral Brett Giroir (video)
Assistant Secretary for Health
Department of Health and Human Services

Huda Akil
Planning Committee Member
University of Michigan

10:00–10:30 am **Audience Discussion**
**Definitions of Brain Health and Resilience**

Moderators: Huda Akil, University of Michigan
Damien Fair, Oregon Health & Science University

10:30 am–12:00 pm **Brain–Body Interactions**

*Driving Questions and Objectives: How does the brain interact with the body, and what implications does this have for measuring and maximizing brain health and resilience? These talks will provide a sample of research on brain–body interactions, demonstrating the importance of this connection and possible avenues for future research on brain health.*

**Colleen McClung, University of Pittsburgh**
Effect of Circadian Rhythms on Health Across the Life Span

**Elinor Sullivan, University of Oregon (remote)**
Early Environmental Risk Factors for Mental Health Disorders

**Natalie Rasgon, Stanford University**
Insulin Resistance—A Link in Brain–Body Interactions

12:00–12:30 pm **Panel and Audience Discussion**
Moderator: Huda Akil, University of Michigan

12:30–1:45 pm **Lunch**

| | |
|---|---|
| 1:45–3:00 pm | **Behavioral and Biological Convergence** |
| | *Driving Questions and Objectives: What are the connections and discontinuities between brain activity and behavior, and between psychological health and brain health? What can behavior and life experience suggest about brain health and resilience? These talks will touch on the biological underpinnings of behavior in the context of cognition, emotion, and psychiatric disorders.* |
| | **Monica Rosenberg, University of Chicago**<br>The Neural Correlates of Attention and Cognition |
| | **Elizabeth Hoge, Georgetown Medical Center**<br>Can Meditation Improve Health and Resilience? |
| 3:00–3:30 pm | **Panel and Audience Discussion**<br>Moderator: Huda Akil, University of Michigan |
| 3:30–3:45 pm | **Break** |
| 3:45–4:30 pm | **Measuring Brain Health** |
| | *Driving Questions and Objectives: What are the methodological techniques and standards for reliability necessary for measuring brain health and resilience? This talk will provide an overview of how quality metrics and criteria can improve measurement of brain health and resilience in future research.* |
| | **Russ Poldrack, Stanford University (remote)**<br>Grand Views and Potholes on the Road to Precision Neuroscience |
| 4:30–5:00 pm | **Panel and Audience Discussion**<br>**The Way Forward in Measurement and Research** |
| | *Objective: Speakers and panelists will reflect on the information presented throughout the day, with a particular focus on generalizable definitions of brain* |

*health and resilience, and how these attributes can be measured.*

Moderator: Huda Akil, University of Michigan

5:00 pm **Adjourn**

**WEDNESDAY, SEPTEMBER 25, 2019**

**Room 125 (note change of Room)**

8:30–8:45 am **Welcome and Overview**
Damien Fair, Oregon Health & Science University

8:45–10:00 am **Brain Health in the Social Context**

*Driving Questions and Objectives: How does an individual's social context affect brain health and resilience? What social factors are most important for understanding and predicting brain health, and how are those factors measured and validated? These talks will provide an overview of brain health in the social context, particularly with respect to emotions and social disparities.*

**Stephanie Cacioppo, University of Chicago**
From Me to We: How Does the Brain Form, Maintain, and Restore Healthy Relationships?

**Gregory Samanez-Larkin, Duke Institute for Brain Sciences (remote)**
Motivation, Cognition, and Decision Making in Everyday Life

**Jennifer Manly, Columbia University Vagelos College of Physicians and Surgeons (remote)**
Life-Course Causes of Later-Life Inequalities in Brain Health

10:00–10:30 am **Panel and Audience Discussion**
Moderator: Damien Fair, Oregon Health & Science University

| | |
|---|---|
| 10:30–10:45 am | **Break** |
| 10:45 am–12:15 pm | **Brain Health Across the Life Span** |

*Driving Questions and Objectives: How do brain health and resilience change across the life span, and how have researchers elected to measure these changes? What do the changes in vulnerabilities and opportunities signal about brain health and resilience at various life stages? These talks will provide an overview of these questions, with a particular focus on typical brain development as well as the development of psychiatric disorders.*

**Deanna Barch, Washington University in St. Louis**
Early Adversity, Emotional Processing, and the Neural Bases of Psychiatric Illness

**Nim Tottenham, Columbia University (remote)**
The Impact of Early-Life Stress on Neurodevelopment

**Ted Satterthwaite, University of Pennsylvania**
Integrating Complex and Personalized Data to Understand Normal and Abnormal Brain Network Development

**Gagan Wig, University of Texas at Dallas**
Brain Network Aging and Health Across the Adult Life Span

| | |
|---|---|
| 12:15–1:00 pm | **Panel and Audience Discussion: The Way Forward in Measurement and Research** |

*Objective: Speakers and panelists will reflect on the information presented throughout the day, with a particular focus on generalizable definitions of brain health and resilience, and how these attributes can be measured.*

Moderator: Damien Fair, Oregon Health & Science University

| | |
|---|---|
| 1:00 pm | **Adjourn** |

# Appendix C

# References


Adam, E. K., L. C. Hawkley, B. M. Kudielka, and J. T. Cacioppo. 2006. Day-to-day dynamics of experience—cortisol associations in a population-based sample of older adults. *Proceedings of the National Academy of Sciences* 103(45):17058–17063.

Adam, K. C. S., I. Mance, K. Fukuda, and E. K. Vogel. 2015. The contribution of attentional lapses to individual differences in visual working memory capacity. *Journal of Cognitive Neuroscience* 27(8):1601–1616.

Adam, K. C. S., M. K. Robison, and E. K. Vogel. 2018. Contralateral delay activity tracks fluctuations in working memory peformance. *Journal of Cognitive Neuroscience* 30(9):1229–1240.

American Psychiatric Association. 2013. *Diagnostic and statistical manual of mental disorders, fifth edition (DSM-5).* Washington, DC: APA.

Aron, A., H. Fisher, D. J. Mashek, G. Strong, H. Li, and L. L. Brown. 2005. Reward, motivation, and emotion systems associated with early-stage intense romantic love. *Journal of Neurophysiology* 94(1):327–337.

Avery, E. W., K. Yoo, M. D. Rosenberg, A. S. Greene, S. Gao, D. L. Na, D. Scheinost, T. R. Constable, and M. M. Chun. 2020. Distributed patterns of functional connectivity predict working memory performance in novel healthy and memory-impaired individuals. *Journal of Cognitive Neuroscience* 32(2):241–255.

Baddeley, A. 1992. Working memory. *Science* 255(5044):556–559.

Barnes, L. L., S. Leurgans, N. T. Aggarwal, R. C. Shah, Z. Arvanitakis, B. D. James, A. S. Buchman, D. A. Bennett, and J. A. Schneider. 2015. Mixed pathology is more likely in black than white decedents with Alzheimer dementia. *Neurology* 85(6):528–534.

Baum, G. L., R. Ciric, D. R. Roalf, R. F. Betzel, T. M. Moore, R. T. Shinohara, A. E. Kahn, S. N. Vandekar, P. E. Rupert, M. Quarmley, P. A. Cook, M. A. Elliott, K. Ruparel, R. E. Gur, R. C. Gur, D. S. Bassett, and T. D. Satterthwaite. 2017. Modular segregation of structural brain networks supports the development of executive function in youth. *Current Biology* 27(11):1561–1572.

Berridge, C. W., D. M. Devilbiss, M. E. Andrzejewski, A. F. Arnsten, A. E. Kelley, B. Schmeichel, C. Hamilton, and R. C. Spencer. 2006. Methylphenidate preferentially increases catecholamine neurotransmission within the prefrontal cortex at low doses that enhance cognitive function. *Biological Psychiatry* 60(10):1111–1120.

Betzel, R. F., L. Byrge, Y. He, J. Goni, X. N. Zuo, and O. Sporns. 2014. Changes in structural and functional connectivity among resting-state networks across the human lifespan. *NeuroImage* 102(2):345–357.

Bigio, B., A. A. Mathé, V. C. Sousa, D. Zelli, P. Svenningsson, B. S. McEwen, and C. Nasca. 2016. Epigenetics and energetics in ventral hippocampus mediate rapid antidepressant action: Implications for treatment resistance. *Proceedings of the National Academy of Sciences* 113(28):7906–7911.

Bijsterbosch, J. D., M. W. Woolrich, M. F. Glasser, E. C. Robinson, C. F. Beckmann, D. C. Van Essen, S. J. Harrison, and S. M. Smith. 2018. The relationship between spatial configuration and functional connectivity of brain regions. *Elife* 7.

Bishop, S. R., M. Lau, S. Shapiro, L. Carlson, N. D. Anderson, J. Carmody, Z. V. Segal, S. Abbey, M. Speca, D. Velting, and G. Devins. 2004. Mindfulness: A proposed operational definition. *Clinical Psychology: Science and Practice* 11(3):230–241.

Bopp, J. M., D. J. Miklowitz, G. M. Goodwin, W. Stevens, J. M. Rendell, and J. R. Geddes. 2010. The longitudinal course of bipolar disorder as revealed through weekly text messaging: A feasibility study. *Bipolar Disorder* 12(3):327–334.

Botvinick-Nezer, R., F. Holzmeister, C. F. Camerer, A. Dreber. J. Huber, M. Johannesson, M. Kirchler, R. Iwanir, J. A. Mumford, A. Adcock, et al. 2019. Variability in the analysis of a single neuroimaging dataset by many teams. bioRxiv, published online November 15.

Bremner, J. D., P. Randall, E. Vermetten, L. Staib, R. A. Bronen, C. Mazure, S. Capelli, G. McCarthy, R. B. Innis, and D. S. Charney. 1997. Magnetic resonance imaging-based measurement of hippocampal volume in posttraumatic stress disorder related to childhood physical and sexual abuse—a preliminary report. *Biological Psychiatry* 41(1):23–32.

Brickman, A. M., N. Schupf, J. J. Manly, J. A. Luchsinger, H. Andrews, M. X. Tang, C. Reitz, S. A. Small, R. Mayeux, C. DeCarli, and T. R. Brown. 2008. Brain morphology in older African Americans, Caribbean Hispanics, and whites from northern Manhattan. *Archives of Neurology* 65(8):1053–1061.

Brown, S. L., D. M. Smith, R. Schulz, M. U. Kabeto, P. A. Ubel, M. Poulin, J. Yi, C. Kim, and K. M. Langa. 2009. Caregiving behavior is associated with decreased mortality risk. *Psychological Science* 20(4):488–494.

Bullmore, E., and O. Sporns. 2009. Complex brain networks: Graph theoretical analysis of structural and functional systems. *Nature Reviews Neuroscience* 10(3):186–198.

Burrows, M., S. M. Rogers, and S. R. Ott. 2011. Epigenetic remodelling of brain, body and behaviour during phase change in locusts. *Neural Systems & Circuits* 1(1):11.

Button, K. S., J. P. A. Ioannidis, C. Mokrysz, B. A. Nosek, J. Flint, E. S. J. Robinson, and M. R. Munafò. 2013. Power failure: Why small sample size undermines the reliability of neuroscience. *Nature Reviews Neuroscience* 14(5):365–376.

Cabeza, R., C. L. Grady, L. Nyberg, A. R. McIntosh, E. Tulving, S. Kapur, J. M. Jennings, S. Houle, and F. I. Craik. 1997. Age-related differences in neural activity during memory encoding and retrieval: A positron emission tomography study. *Journal of Neuroscience* 17(1):391–400.

Cacioppo, J. T., and S. Cacioppo. 2012. The phenotype of loneliness. *European Journal of Developmental Psychology* 9(4):446–452.

Cacioppo, J. T., and S. Cacioppo. 2014. Social relationships and health: The toxic effects of perceived social isolation. *Social and Personality Psychology Compass* 8(2):58–72.

Cacioppo, J. T., and S. Cacioppo. 2018a. The growing problem of loneliness. *Lancet* 391(10119):426.

Cacioppo, J. T., and S. Cacioppo. 2018b. Loneliness in the modern age: An evolutionary theory of loneliness. In *Advances in experimental social psychology*. Vol. 58, edited by J. M. Olson. Cambridge, MA: Academic Press. Pp. 127–197.

Cacioppo, J. T., and W. Patrick. 2008. Loneliness: Human nature and the need for social connection. *The Wall Street Journal*. November 28.

Cacioppo, J. T., J. M. Ernst, M. H. Burleson, M. K. McClintock, W. B. Malarkey, L. C. Hawkley, R. B. Kowalewski, A. Paulsen, J. A. Hobson, K. Hugdahl, D. Spiegel, and G. G. Berntson. 2000. Lonely traits and concomitant physiological processes: The Macarthur social neuroscience studies. *International Journal of Psychophysiology* 35(2–3):143–154.

Cacioppo, J. T., L. C. Hawkley, G. G. Berntson, J. M. Ernst, A. C. Gibbs, R. Stickgold, and J. A. Hobson. 2002a. Do lonely days invade the nights? Potential social modulation of sleep efficiency. *Psychological Science* 13(4):384–387.

Cacioppo, J. T., L. C. Hawkley, L. E. Crawford, J. M. Ernst, M. H. Burleson, R. B. Kowalewski, W. B. Malarkey, E. Van Cauter, and G. G. Berntson. 2002b. Loneliness and health: Potential mechanisms. *Psychosomatic Medicine* 64(3):407–417.

Cacioppo, J. T., M. E. Hughes, L. J. Waite, L. C. Hawkley, and R. A. Thisted. 2006. Loneliness as a specific risk factor for depressive symptoms: Cross-sectional and longitudinal analyses. *Psychology of Aging* 21(1):140–151.

Cacioppo, J. T., C. J. Norris, J. Decety, G. Monteleone, and H. Nusbaum. 2009. In the eye of the beholder: Individual differences in perceived social isolation predict regional brain activation to social stimuli. *Journal of Cognitive Neuroscience* 21(1):83–92.

Cacioppo, J. T., L. C. Hawkley, and R. A. Thisted. 2010. Perceived social isolation makes me sad: 5-year cross-lagged analyses of loneliness and depressive symptomatology in the Chicago health, aging, and social relations study. *Psychology and Aging* 25(2):453–463.

Cacioppo, J. T., H. T. Reis, and A. J. Zautra. 2011. Social resilience: The value of social fitness with an application to the military. *American Psychology* 66(1):43–51.

Cacioppo, S. 2018. Neuroscience of salutary close relationships. In *The Cambridge handbook of personal relationships*, 2nd ed. Cambridge, MA: Cambridge University Press.

Cacioppo, S., C. Frum, E. Asp, R. M. Weiss, J. W. Lewis, and J. T. Cacioppo. 2013. A quantitative meta-analysis of functional imaging studies of social rejection. *Scientific Reports* 3:2027.

Cacioppo, S., J. P. Capitanio, and J. T. Cacioppo. 2014. Toward a neurology of loneliness. *Psychological Bulletin* 140(6):1464–1504.

Cacioppo, S., S. Balogh, and J. T. Cacioppo. 2015a. Implicit attention to negative social, in contrast to nonsocial, words in the Stroop task differs between individuals high and low in loneliness: Evidence from event-related brain microstates. *Cortex* 70:213–233.

Cacioppo, S., A. J. Grippo, S. London, L. Goossens, and J. T. Cacioppo. 2015b. Loneliness: Clinical import and interventions. *Perspectives on Psychological Science* 10(2):238–249.

Cacioppo, S., M. Bangee, S. Balogh, C. Cardenas-Iniguez, P. Qualter, and J. T. Cacioppo. 2016. Loneliness and implicit attention to social threat: A high-performance electrical neuroimaging study. *Journal of Cognitive Neuroscience* 7(1–4):138–159.

Callaghan, B. L., and N. Tottenham. 2016. The stress acceleration hypothesis: Effects of early-life adversity on emotion circuits and behavior. *Current Opinion in Behavioral Sciences* 7:76–81.

Carp, J. 2012. On the plurality of (methodological) worlds: Estimating the analytic flexibility of fMRI experiments. *Frontiers in Neuroscience* 6:149.

Carrión, V. G., B. W. Haas, A. Garrett, S. Song, and A. L. Reiss. 2010. Reduced hippocampal activity in youth with posttraumatic stress symptoms: An fMRI study. *Journal of Pediatric Psychology* 35(5):559–569.

Carstensen, L. L., and B. L. Fredrickson. 1998. Influence of HIV status and age on cognitive representations of others. *Health and Psychology* 17(6):494–503.

Cassady, K., H. Gagnon, P. Lalwani, M. Simmonite, B. Foerster, D. Park, S. J. Peltier, M. Petrou, S. F. Taylor, D. H. Weissman, R. D. Seidler, and T. A. Polk. 2019. Sensorimotor network segregation declines with age and is linked to GABA and to sensorimotor performance. *NeuroImage* 186:234–244.

Chan, M. Y., D. C. Park, N. K. Savalia, S. E. Petersen, and G. S. Wig. 2014. Decreased segregation of brain systems across the healthy adult lifespan. *Proceedings of the National Academy of Sciences* 111(46):E4997–E5006.

Chan, M. Y., J. Na, P. F. Agres, N. K. Savalia, D. C. Park, and G. S. Wig. 2018. Socioeconomic status moderates age-related differences in the brain's functional network organization and anatomy across the adult lifespan. *Proceedings of the National Academy of Sciences* 15(22):E5144–E5153.

Chauhan, R., K.-F. Chen, B. A. Kent, and D. C. Crowther. 2017. Central and peripheral circadian clocks and their role in Alzheimer's disease. *Disease Models & Mechanisms* 10(10):1187–1199.

Chong, J. S. X., K. K. Ng, J. Tandi, C. Wang, J.-H. Poh, J. C. Lo, M. W. L. Chee, and J. H. Zhou. 2019. Longitudinal changes in the cerebral cortex functional organization of healthy elderly. *Journal of Neuroscience* 39(28):5534–5550.

Christoff, K., A. M. Gordon, J. Smallwood, R. Smith, and J. W. Schooler. 2009. Experience sampling during fMRI reveals default network and executive system contributions to mind wandering. *Proceedings of the National Academy of Sciences* 106(21):8719.

Coelho, Jr., A. M., K. D. Carey, and R. E. Shade. 1991. Assessing the effects of social environment on blood pressure and heart rates of baboons. *American Journal of Primatology* 23(4):257–267.

Cohen, M. R., and J. H. R. Maunsell. 2011. When attention wanders: How uncontrolled fluctuations in attention affect performance. *Journal of Neuroscience* 31(44):15802.

Cole, S. W., L. C. Hawkley, J. M. Arevalo, C. Y. Sung, R. M. Rose, and J. T. Cacioppo. 2007. Social regulation of gene expression in human leukocytes. *Genome Biology* 8(9):R189.

Cole, S. W., L. C. Hawkley, J. M. G. Arevalo, and J. T. Cacioppo. 2011. Transcript origin analysis identifies antigen-presenting cells as primary targets of socially regulated gene expression in leukocytes. *Proceedings of the National Academy of Sciences* 108(7):3080–3085.

Cole, S. W., M. E. Levine, J. M. G. Arevalo, J. Ma, D. R. Weir, and E. M. Crimmins. 2015. Loneliness, eudaimonia, and the human conserved transcriptional response to adversity. *Psychoneuroendocrinology* 62:11–17.

Copas, J. B. 1983. Regression, prediction and shrinkage. *Journal of the Royal Statistical Society. Series B (Methodological)* 45(3):311–354.

Cui, Z., H. Li, C. H. Xia, B. Larsen, A. Adebimpe, G. L. Baum, M. Cieslak, R. E. Gur, R. C. Gur, T. M. Moore, D. J. Oathes, A. F. Alexander-Bloch, A. Raznahan, D. R. Roalf, R. T. Shinohara, D. H. Wolf, C. Davatzikos, D. S. Bassett, D. A. Fair, Y. Fan, and T. D. Satterthwaite. 2020. Individual variation in functional topography of association networks in youth. *Neuron*, February 11. [Epub ahead of print].

Darki, F., and T. Klingberg. 2015. The role of fronto-parietal and fronto-striatal networks in the development of working memory: A longitudinal study. *Cerebral Cortex* 25(6):1587–1595.

Davidson, J. R., V. M. Payne, K. M. Connor, E. B. Foa, B. O. Rothbaum, M. A. Hertzberg, and R. H. Weisler. 2005. Trauma, resilience and saliostasis: Effects of treatment in posttraumatic stress disorder. *International Clinical Psychopharmacology* 20(1):43–48.

deBettencourt, M. T., J. D. Cohen, R. F. Lee, K. A. Norman, and N. B. Turk-Browne. 2015. Closed-loop training of attention with real-time brain imaging. *Nature Neuroscience* 18(3):470–475.

deBettencourt, M. T., K. A. Norman, and N. B. Turk-Browne. 2018. Forgetting from lapses of sustained attention. *Psychonomic Bulletin & Review* 25(2):605–611.

Dinga, R., L. Schmaal, B. W. J. H. Penninx, M. J. van Tol, D. J. Veltman, L. van Velzen, M. Mennes, N. J. A. van der Wee, and A. F. Marquand. 2019. Evaluating the evidence for biotypes of depression: Methodological replication and extension of. *NeuroImage: Clinical* 22:101796.

Driessen, M., J. Herrmann, K. Stahl, M. Zwaan, S. Meier, A. Hill, M. Osterheider, and D. Petersen. 2000. Magnetic resonance imaging volumes of the hippocampus and the amygdala in women with borderline personality disorder and early traumatization. *Archives of General Psychiatry* 57(12):1115–1122.

Drysdale, A. T., L. Grosenick, J. Downar, K. Dunlop, F. Mansouri, Y. Meng, R. N. Fetcho, B. Zebley, D. J. Oathes, A. Etkin, A. F. Schatzberg, K. Sudheimer, J. Keller, H. S. Mayberg, F. M. Gunning, G. S. Alexopoulos, M. D. Fox, A. Pascual-Leone, H. U. Voss, B. J. Casey, M. J. Dubin, and C. Liston. 2016. Resting-state connectivity biomarkers define neurophysiological subtypes of depression. *Nature Medicine* 23:28.

Edmiston, E. E., F. Wang, C. M. Mazure, J. Guiney, R. Sinha, L. C. Mayes, and H. P. Blumberg. 2011. Corticostriatal-limbic gray matter morphology in adolescents with self-reported exposure to childhood maltreatment. *Archives of Pediatric and Adolescent Medicine* 165(12):1069–1077.

Edmondson, B. 2010. All the lonely people. *AARP* 83. *The Magazine*, November/December issue.

Epel, E. S., E. H. Blackburn, J. Lin, F. S. Dhabhar, N. E. Adler, J. D. Morrow, and R. M. Cawthon. 2004. Accelerated telomere shortening in response to life stress. *Proceedings of the National Academy of Sciences* 101(49):17312–17315.

Esterman, M., S. K. Noonan, M. Rosenberg, and J. Degutis. 2013. In the zone or zoning out? Tracking behavioral and neural fluctuations during sustained attention. *Cerebral Cortex* 23(11):2712–2723.

Fair, D. A., N. U. Dosenbach, J. A. Church, A. L. Cohen, S. Brahmbhatt, F. M. Miezin, D. M. Barch, M. E. Raichle, S. E. Petersen, and B. L. Schlaggar. 2007. Development of distinct control networks through segregation and integration. *Proceedings of the National Academy of Sciences* 104(33):13507–13512.

Farr, O. M., S. Hu, D. Matuskey, S. Zhang, O. Abdelghany, and C.-S. R. Li. 2014a. The effects of methylphenidate on cerebral activations to salient stimuli in healthy adults. *Experimental and Clinical Psychopharmacology* 22(2):154–165.

Farr, O. M., S. Zhang, S. Hu, D. Matuskey, O. Abdelghany, R. T. Malison, and C.-S. R. Li. 2014b. The effects of methylphenidate on resting-state striatal, thalamic and global functional connectivity in healthy adults. *International Journal of Neuropsychopharmacology* 17(8):1177–1191.

Finn, E. S., X. Shen, D. Scheinost, M. D. Rosenberg, J. Huang, M. M. Chun, X. Papademetris, and R. T. Constable. 2015. Functional connectome fingerprinting: Identifying individuals using patterns of brain connectivity. *Nature Neuroscience* 18(11):1664–1671.

Finn, E. S., D. Scheinost, D. M. Finn, X. Shen, X. Papademetris, and R. T. Constable. 2017. Can brain state be manipulated to emphasize individual differences in functional connectivity? *NeuroImage* 160:140–151.

Fish, E. W., D. Shahrokh, R. Bagot, C. Caldji, T. Bredy, M. Szyf, and M. J. Meaney. 2004. Epigenetic programming of stress responses through variations in maternal care. *Annals of the New York Academy of Science* 1036:167–180.

Fredrickson, B. L., and L. L. Carstensen. 1990. Choosing social partners: How old age and anticipated endings make people more selective. *Psychology and Aging* 5(3):335–347.

Fung, H. H., L. L. Carstensen, and A. M. Lutz. 1999. Influence of time on social preferences: Implications for life-span development. *Psychology and Aging* 14(4):595–604.

Gabard-Durnam, L. J., and K. A. McLaughlin. 2019. Do sensitive periods exist for exposure to adversity? *Biological Psychiatry* 85(10):789–791.

Gabard-Durnam, L. J., J. Flannery, B. Goff, D. G. Gee, K. L. Humphreys, E. Telzer, T. Hare, and N. Tottenham. 2014. The development of human amygdala functional connectivity at rest from 4 to 23 years: A cross-sectional study. *NeuroImage* 95:193–207.

Gabard-Durnam, L. J., D. G. Gee, B. Goff, J. Flannery, E. Telzer, K. L. Humphreys, D. S. Lumian, D. S. Fareri, C. Caldera, and N. Tottenham. 2016. Stimulus-elicited connectivity influences resting-state connectivity years later in human development: A prospective study. *Journal of Neuroscience* 36(17):4771–4784.

Gard, T., M. Taquet, R. Dixit, B. K. Hölzel, Y.-A. de Montjoye, N. Brach, D. H. Salat, B. C. Dickerson, J. R. Gray, and S. W. Lazar. 2014. Fluid intelligence and brain functional organization in aging yoga and meditation practitioners. *Frontiers in Aging Neuroscience* 6:76.

Gee, D. G., L. J. Gabard-Durnam, J. Flannery, B. Goff, K. L. Humphreys, E. H. Telzer, T. A. Hare, S. Y. Bookheimer, and N. Tottenham. 2013a. Early developmental emergence of human amygdala–prefrontal connectivity after maternal deprivation. *Proceedings of the National Academy of Sciences* 110(39):15638–15643.

Gee, D. G., K. L. Humphreys, J. Flannery, B. Goff, E. H. Telzer, M. Shapiro, T. A. Hare, S. Y. Bookheimer, and N. Tottenham. 2013b. A developmental shift from positive to negative connectivity in human amygdala–prefrontal circuitry. *Journal of Neuroscience* 33(10):4584–4593.

Gee, D. G., L. Gabard-Durnam, E. H. Telzer, K. L. Humphreys, B. Goff, M. Shapiro, J. Flannery, D. S. Lumian, D. S. Fareri, C. Caldera, and N. Tottenham. 2014. Maternal buffering of human amygdala-prefrontal circuitry during childhood but not during adolescence. *Psychological Science* 25(11):2067–2078.

Geerligs, L., R. J. Renken, E. Saliasi, N. M. Maurits, and M. M. Lorist. 2014. A brain-wide study of age-related changes in functional connectivity. *Cerebral Cortex* 25(7):1987–1999.

Glymour, M. M., A. Kosheleva, V. G. Wadley, C. Weiss, and J. J. Manly. 2011. Geographic distribution of dementia mortality: Elevated mortality rates for black and white Americans by place of birth. *Alzheimer Disease and Associated Disorders* 25(3):196–202.

Goodwin, J. S., W. C. Hunt, C. R. Key, and J. M. Samet. 1987. The effect of marital status on stage, treatment, and survival of cancer patients. *JAMA* 258(21):3125–3130.

Goossens, N., S. Nakagawa, X. Sun, and Y. Hoshida. 2015. Cancer biomarker discovery and validation. *Translational Cancer Research* 4(3):256–269.

Gordon, E. M., T. O. Laumann, A. W. Gilmore, D. J. Newbold, D. J. Greene, J. J. Berg, M. Ortega, C. Hoyt-Drazen, C. Gratton, H. Sun, J. M. Hampton, R. S. Coalson, A. L. Nguyen, K. B. McDermott, J. S. Shimony, A. Z. Snyder, B. L. Schlaggar, S. E. Petersen, S. M. Nelson, and N. U. F. Dosenbach. 2017. Precision functional mapping of individual human brains. *Neuron* 95(4):791–807.

Gotlib, I. H., J. LeMoult, N. L. Colich, L. C. Foland-Ross, J. Hallmayer, J. Joormann, J. Lin, and O. M. Wolkowitz. 2015. Telomere length and cortisol reactivity in children of depressed mothers. *Molecular Psychiatry* 20(5):615–620.

Grady, C., S. Sarraf, C. Saverino, and K. Campbell. 2016. Age differences in the functional interactions among the default, frontoparietal control, and dorsal attention networks. *Neurobiology and Aging* 41:159–172.

Greenhill, L. L., R. L. Findling, and J. M. Swanson. 2002. A double-blind, placebo-controlled study of modified-release methylphenidate in children with attention-deficit/hyperactivity disorder. *Pediatrics* 109(3):E39.

Grippo, A. J., E. Ihm, J. Wardwell, N. McNeal, M. A. Scotti, D. A. Moenk, D. L. Chandler, M. A. LaRocca, and K. Preihs. 2014. The effects of environmental enrichment on depressive and anxiety-relevant behaviors in socially isolated prairie voles. *Psychosomatic Medicine* 76(4):277–284.

Grivas, T. B., and O. D. Savvidou. 2007. Melatonin the "light of night" in human biology and adolescent idiopathic scoliosis. *Scoliosis* 2(1):6.

Gustafsson, H. C., K. F. Holton, A. N. Anderson, E. K. Nousen, C. A. Sullivan, J. M. Loftis, J. T. Nigg, and E. L. Sullivan. 2019. Increased maternal prenatal adiposity, inflammation, and lower omega-3 fatty acid levels influence child negative affect. *Frontiers in Neuroscience* 13:1035.

Han, L., N. K. Savalia, M. Y. Chan, P. F. Agres, A. S. Nair, and G. S. Wig. 2018. Functional parcellation of the cerebral cortex across the human adult lifespan. *Cerebral Cortex* 28(12):4403–4423.

Hanson, J. L., A. R. Knodt, B. D. Brigidi, and A. R. Hariri. 2015. Lower structural integrity of the uncinate fasciculus is associated with a history of child maltreatment and future psychological vulnerability to stress. *Development and Psychopathology* 27(4 Pt 2):1611–1619.

Hasler, B. P., S. L. Sitnick, D. S. Shaw, and E. E. Forbes. 2013. An altered neural response to reward may contribute to alcohol problems among late adolescents with an evening chronotype. *Psychiatry Research* 214(3):357–364.

Hatori, M., C. Vollmers, A. Zarrinpar, L. DiTacchio, E. A. Bushong, S. Gill, M. Leblanc, A. Chaix, M. Joens, J. A. Fitzpatrick, M. H. Ellisman, and S. Panda. 2012. Time-restricted feeding without reducing caloric intake prevents metabolic diseases in mice fed a high-fat diet. *Cell Metabolism* 15(6):848–860.

Hawkley, L. C., K. J. Preacher, and J. T. Cacioppo. 2010a. Loneliness impairs daytime functioning but not sleep duration. *Health and Psychology* 29(2):124–129.

Hawkley, L. C., R. A. Thisted, C. M. Masi, and J. T. Cacioppo. 2010b. Loneliness predicts increased blood pressure: 5-year cross-lagged analyses in middle-aged and older adults. *Psychology and Aging* 25(1):132–141.

Hofmann, S. G., and P. M. Dibartolo. 2000. An instrument to assess self-statements during public speaking: Scale development and preliminary psychometric properties. *Behavioral Therapy* 31(3):499–515.

Hoge, E. A., E. Bui, L. Marques, C. A. Metcalf, L. K. Morris, D. J. Robinaugh, J. J. Worthington, M. H. Pollack, and N. M. Simon. 2013a. Randomized controlled trial of mindfulness meditation for generalized anxiety disorder: Effects on anxiety and stress reactivity. *Journal of Clinical Psychiatry* 74(8):786–792.

Hoge, E. A., M. M. Chen, E. Orr, C. A. Metcalf, L. E. Fischer, M. H. Pollack, I. De Vivo, and N. M. Simon. 2013b. Loving-kindness meditation practice associated with longer telomeres in women. *Brain, Behavior, and Immunity* 32:159–163.

Hohman, T. J., J. N. Cooke-Bailey, C. Reitz, G. Jun, A. Naj, G. W. Beecham, Z. Liu, R. M. Carney, J. M. Vance, M. L. Cuccaro, R. Rajbhandary, B. N. Vardarajan, L. S. Wang, O. Valladares, C. F. Lin, E. B. Larson, N. R. Graff-Radford, D. Evans, P. L. De Jager, P. K. Crane, J. D. Buxbaum, J. R. Murrell, T. Raj, N. Ertekin-Taner, M. W. Logue, C. T. Baldwin, R. C. Green, L. L. Barnes, L. B. Cantwell, M. D. Fallin, R. C. Go, P. Griffith, T. O. Obisesan, J. J. Manly, K. L. Lunetta, M. I. Kamboh, O. L. Lopez, D. A. Bennett, J. Hardy, H. C. Hendrie, K. S. Hall, A. M. Goate, R. Lang, G. S. Byrd, W. A. Kukull, T. M. Foroud, L. A. Farrer, E. R. Martin, M. A. Pericak-Vance, G. D. Schellenberg, R. Mayeux, J. L. Haines, and T. A. Thornton-Wells. 2016. Global and local ancestry in African-Americans: Implications for Alzheimer's disease risk. *Alzheimer's & Dementia* 12(3):233–243.

Holland, C. A. C., N. C. Ebner, T. Lin, and G. R. Samanez-Larkin. 2019. Emotion identification across adulthood using the dynamic faces database of emotional expressions in younger, middle aged, and older adults. *Cognition and Emotion* 33(2):245–257.

Holmes, A. J., and L. M. Patrick. 2018. The myth of optimality in clinical neuroscience. *Trends in Cognitive Sciences* 22(3):241–257.

Holt-Lunstad, J., T. B. Smith, and J. B. Layton. 2010. Social relationships and mortality risk: A meta-analytic review. *PLoS Medicine* 7(7):e1000316.

Hölzel, B. K., E. A. Hoge, D. N. Greve, T. Gard, J. D. Creswell, K. W. Brown, L. F. Barrett, C. Schwartz, D. Vaitl, and S. W. Lazar. 2013. Neural mechanisms of symptom improvements in generalized anxiety disorder following mindfulness training. *NeuroImage: Clinical* 2:448–458.

Howard, V. J., D. O. Kleindorfer, S. E. Judd, L. A. McClure, M. M. Safford, J. D. Rhodes, M. Cushman, C. S. Moy, E. Z. Soliman, B. M. Kissela, and G. Howard. 2011. Disparities in stroke incidence contributing to disparities in stroke mortality. *Annals of Neurology* 69(4):619–627.

Huang, A. R., K. L. Strombotne, E. M. Horner, and S. J. Lapham. 2018. Adolescent cognitive aptitudes and later-in-life Alzheimer disease and related disorders. *JAMA Network Open* 1(5):e181726.

Ioannidis, J. P. A. 2005. Why most published research findings are false. *PLoS Medicine* 2(8):e124.

Jaremka, L. M., C. P. Fagundes, J. Peng, J. M. Bennett, R. Glaser, W. B. Malarkey, and J. K. Kiecolt-Glaser. 2013. Loneliness promotes inflammation during acute stress. *Psychological Science* 24(7):1089–1097.

Johansson, A.-S., J. Brask, B. Owe-Larsson, J. Hetta, and G. B. S. Lundkvist. 2011. Valproic acid phase shifts the rhythmic expression of PERIOD2::LUCIFERASE. *Journal of Biological Rhythms* 26(6):541–551.

Kane, M. J., and R. W. Engle. 2002. The role of prefrontal cortex in working-memory capacity, executive attention, and general fluid intelligence: An individual-differences perspective. *Psychonomic Bulletin & Review* 9(4):637–671.

Kaplan, R. M., and V. L. Irvin. 2015. Likelihood of null effects of large NHLBI clinical trials has increased over time. *PLoS One* 10(8):e0132382.

Karelina, K., G. J. Norman, N. Zhang, J. S. Morris, H. Peng, and A. C. DeVries. 2009. Social isolation alters neuroinflammatory response to stroke. *Proceedings of the National Academy of Sciences* 106(14):5895–5900.

Karrer, T. M., A. K. Josef, R. Mata, E. D. Morris, and G. R. Samanez-Larkin. 2017. Reduced dopamine receptors and transporters but not synthesis capacity in normal aging adults: A meta-analysis. *Neurobiology and Aging* 57:36–46.

Kasper, D. L., A. S. Fauci, S. L. Hauser, D. L. Longo, J. L. Jameson, and J. Loscalzo. 2018. *Harrison's principles of internal medicine*. Vol. 1, 2. New York: McGraw-Hill Professional.

Kaushal, N., V. Ramesh, and D. Gozal. 2012. TNF-α and temporal changes in sleep architecture in mice exposed to sleep fragmentation. *PLoS One* 7(9):e45610.

Kenna, H., F. Hoeft, R. Kelley, T. Wroolie, B. DeMuth, A. Reiss, and N. Rasgon. 2013. Fasting plasma insulin and the default mode network in women at risk for Alzheimer's disease. *Neurobiology of Aging* 34(3):641–649.

Kessler, R. C., K. A. McLaughlin, J. G. Green, M. J. Gruber, N. A. Sampson, A. M. Zaslavsky, S. Aguilar-Gaxiola, A. O. Alhamzawi, J. Alonso, M. Angermeyer, C. Benjet, E. Bromet, S. Chatterji, G. de Girolamo, K. Demyttenaere, J. Fayyad, S. Florescu, G. Gal, O. Gureje, J. M. Haro, C. Y. Hu, E. G. Karam, N. Kawakami, S. Lee, J. P. Lepine, J. Ormel, J. Posada-Villa, R. Sagar, A. Tsang, T. B. Ustun, S. Vassilev, M. C. Viana, and D. R. Williams. 2010. Childhood adversities and adult psychopathology in the WHO world mental health surveys. *British Journal of Psychiatry* 197(5):378–385.

Keyes, K. M., and D. Westreich. 2019. UK biobank, big data, and the consequences of non-representativeness. *Lancet* 393(10178):1297.

King, B. R., P. van Ruitenbeek, I. Leunissen, K. Cuypers, K.-F. Heise, T. Santos Monteiro, L. Hermans, O. Levin, G. Albouy, D. Mantini, and S. P. Swinnen. 2017. Age-related declines in motor performance are associated with decreased segregation of large-scale resting state brain networks. *Cerebral Cortex* 28(12):4390–4402.

Klingberg, T., H. Forssberg, and H. Westerberg. 2002. Training of working memory in children with ADHD. *Journal of Clinical and Experimental Neuropsychology* 24(6):781–791.

Kohsaka, A., A. D. Laposky, K. M. Ramsey, C. Estrada, C. Joshu, Y. Kobayashi, F. W. Turek, and J. Bass. 2007. High-fat diet disrupts behavioral and molecular circadian rhythms in mice. *Cell Metabolism* 6(5):414–421.

Kong, R., J. Li, C. Orban, M. R. Sabuncu, H. Liu, A. Schaefer, N. Sun, X. N. Zuo, A. J. Holmes, S. B. Eickhoff, and B. T. T. Yeo. 2019. Spatial topography of individual-specific cortical networks predicts human cognition, personality, and emotion. *Cerebral Cortex* 29(6):2533–2551.

Koster, A., B. W. Penninx, H. Bosma, G. I. Kempen, A. B. Newman, S. M. Rubin, S. Satterfield, H. H. Atkinson, H. N. Ayonayon, C. Rosano, K. Yaffe, T. B. Harris, R. N. Rooks, J. T. Van Eijk, and S. B. Kritchevsky. 2005. Socioeconomic differences in cognitive decline and the role of biomedical factors. *Annals of Epidemiology* 15(8):564–571.

Kupper, Z., and H. Hoffmann. 2000. Course patterns of psychosocial functioning in schizophrenia patients attending a vocational rehabilitation program. *Schizophrenia Bulletin* 26(3):681–698.

Lake, E. M. R., E. S. Finn, S. M. Noble, T. Vanderwal, X. Shen, M. D. Rosenberg, M. N. Spann, M. M. Chun, D. Scheinost, and R. T. Constable. 2019. The functional brain organization of an individual allows prediction of measures of social abilities transdiagnostically in autism and attention-deficit/hyperactivity disorder. *Biological Psychiatry* 86(4):315–326.

Laumann, T. O., E. M. Gordon, B. Adeyemo, A. Z. Snyder, S. J. Joo, M.-Y. Chen, A. W. Gilmore, K. B. McDermott, S. M. Nelson, N. U. F. Dosenbach, B. L. Schlaggar, J. A. Mumford, R. A. Poldrack, and S. E. Petersen. 2015. Functional system and areal organization of a highly sampled individual human brain. *Neuron* 87(3):657–670.

Lazar, S. W., C. E. Kerr, R. H. Wasserman, J. R. Gray, D. N. Greve, M. T. Treadway, M. McGarvey, B. T. Quinn, J. A. Dusek, H. Benson, S. L. Rauch, C. I. Moore, and B. Fischl. 2005. Meditation experience is associated with increased cortical thickness. *NeuroReport* 16(17):1893–1897.

Lee, F. S., H. Heimer, J. N. Giedd, E. S. Lein, N. Sestan, D. R. Weinberger, and B. J. Casey. 2014. Adolescent mental health—Opportunity and obligation. *Science* 346(6209):547–549.

Levi, F., C. Focan, A. Karaboue, V. de la Valette, D. Focan-Henrard, B. Baron, F. Kreutz, and S. Giacchetti. 2007. Implications of circadian clocks for the rhythmic delivery of cancer therapeutics. *Advanced Drug Delivery Reviews* 59(9–10):1015–1035.

Li, J., W.-Q. Lu, S. Beesley, A. S. I. Loudon, and Q.-J. Meng. 2012. Lithium impacts on the amplitude and period of the molecular circadian clockwork. *PLoS One* 7(3):e33292.

Li, J., W. Han, K. A. Pelkey, J. Duan, X. Mao, Y. X. Wang, M. T. Craig, L. Dong, R. S. Petralia, C. J. McBain, and W. Lu. 2017. Molecular dissection of Neuroligin 2 and Slitrk3 reveals an essential framework for GABAergic synapse development. *Neuron* 96(4):808–826.

Li, X., J. Q. Gan, and H. Wang. 2018. Collective sparse symmetric non-negative matrix factorization for identifying overlapping communities in resting-state brain functional networks. *NeuroImage* 166:259–275.

Lillard, L. A., M. J. Brien, and L. J. Waite. 1995. Premarital cohabitation and subsequent marital dissolution: A matter of self-selection? *Demography* 32(3):437–457.

Lin, K. W., T. E. Wroolie, T. Robakis, and N. L. Rasgon. 2015. Adjuvant pioglitazone for unremitted depression: Clinical correlates of treatment response. *Psychiatry Research* 230(3):846–852.

Liston, C., M. M. Miller, D. S. Goldwater, J. J. Radley, A. B. Rocher, P. R. Hof, J. H. Morrison, and B. S. McEwen. 2006. Stress-induced alterations in prefrontal cortical dendritic morphology predict selective impairments in perceptual attentional set-shifting. *Journal of Neuroscience* 26(30):7870–7874.

Liu, D., J. Diorio, B. Tannenbaum, C. Caldji, D. Francis, A. Freedman, S. Sharma, D. Pearson, P. M. Plotsky, and M. J. Meaney. 1997. Maternal care, hippocampal glucocorticoid receptors, and hypothalamic-pituitary-adrenal responses to stress. *Science* 277(5332):1659–1662.

Logan, R. W., and C. A. McClung. 2019. Rhythms of life: Circadian disruption and brain disorders across the lifespan. *Nature Reviews Neuroscience* 20(1):49–65.

Logan, R. W., C. Zhang, S. Murugan, S. O'Connell, D. Levitt, A. M. Rosenwasser, and D. K. Sarkar. 2012. Chronic shift-lag alters the circadian clock of NK cells and promotes lung cancer growth in rats. *Journal of Immunology* 188(6):2583.

Long, J. E., M. T. Drayson, A. E. Taylor, K. M. Toellner, J. M. Lord, and A. C. Phillips. 2016. Morning vaccination enhances antibody response over afternoon vaccination: A cluster-randomised trial. *Vaccine* 34(24):2679–2685.

Luby, J. L., A. Belden, M. P. Harms, R. Tillman, and D. M. Barch. 2016. Preschool is a sensitive period for the influence of maternal support on the trajectory of hippocampal development. *Proceedings of the National Academy of Sciences* 113(20):5742–5747.

Luo, Y., L. C. Hawkley, L. J. Waite, and J. T. Cacioppo. 2012. Loneliness, health, and mortality in old age: A national longitudinal study. *Social Science and Medicine* 74(6):907–914.

Lutz, A., H. A. Slagter, J. D. Dunne, and R. J. Davidson. 2008. Attention regulation and monitoring in meditation. *Trends in Cognitive Sciences* 12(4):163–169.

Magarinos, A. M., and B. S. McEwen. 1995. Stress-induced atrophy of apical dendrites of hippocampal ca3c neurons: Involvement of glucocorticoid secretion and excitatory amino acid receptors. *Neuroscience* 69(1):89–98.

Marden, J. R., S. Walter, J. S. Kaufman, and M. M. Glymour. 2016. African ancestry, social factors, and hypertension among non-hispanic blacks in the health and retirement study. *Biodemography and Social Biology* 62(1):19–35.

Maslowsky, J., K. Mogg, B. P. Bradley, E. McClure-Tone, M. Ernst, D. S. Pine, and C. S. Monk. 2010. A preliminary investigation of neural correlates of treatment in adolescents with generalized anxiety disorder. *Journal of Child and Adolescent Psychopharmacology* 20(2):105–111.

Matsumoto, K., K. Ono, H. Ouchi, R. Tsushima, and Y. Murakami. 2012. Social isolation stress down-regulates cortical early growth response 1 (EGR-1) expression in mice. *Neuroscience Research* 73(3):257–262.

Mayeda, E. R., M. M. Glymour, C. P. Quesenberry, and R. A. Whitmer. 2016. Inequalities in dementia incidence between six racial and ethnic groups over 14 years. *Alzheimer's & Dementia* 12(3):216–224.

McDermott, C. L., J. Seidlitz, A. Nadig, S. Liu, L. S. Clasen, J. D. Blumenthal, P. K. Reardon, F. Lalonde, D. Greenstein, R. Patel, M. M. Chakravarty, J. P. Lerch, and A. Raznahan. 2019. Longitudinally mapping childhood socioeconomic status associations with cortical and subcortical morphology. *Journal of Neuroscience* 39(8):1365–1373.

McIntyre, R. S., N. L. Rasgon, D. E. Kemp, H. T. Nguyen, C. W. Law, V. H. Taylor, H. O. Woldeyohannes, M. T. Alsuwaidan, J. K. Soczynska, B. Kim, M. T. Lourenco, L. S. Kahn, and B. I. Goldstein. 2009. Metabolic syndrome and major depressive disorder: Co-occurrence and pathophysiologic overlap. *Current Diabetes Reports* 9(1):51–59.

Meaney, M. J. 2001. Maternal care, gene expression, and the transmission of individual differences in stress reactivity across generations. *Annual Review of Neuroscience* 24:1161–1192.

Mendoza, S. P., and W. A. Mason. 1986. Contrasting responses to intruders and to involuntary separation by monogamous and polygynous New World monkeys. *Physiology and Behavior* 38(6):795–801.

Mennin, D. S., D. M. Fresco, R. G. Heimberg, F. R. Schneier, S. O. Davies, and M. R. Liebowitz. 2002. Screening for social anxiety disorder in the clinical setting: Using the Liebowitz social anxiety scale. *Journal of Anxiety Disorders* 16(6):661–673.

Mennin, D. S., R. G. Heimberg, C. L. Turk, and D. M. Fresco. 2005. Preliminary evidence for an emotion dysregulation model of generalized anxiety disorder. *Behavior Research and Therapy* 43(10):1281–1310.

Miranda-Dominguez, O., B. D. Mills, S. D. Carpenter, K. A. Grant, C. D. Kroenke, J. T. Nigg, and D. A. Fair. 2014. Connectotyping: Model based fingerprinting of the functional connectome. *PLoS One* 9(11):e111048.

Mitra, R., S. Jadhav, B. S. McEwen, A. Vyas, and S. Chattarji. 2005. Stress duration modulates the spatiotemporal patterns of spine formation in the basolateral amygdala. *Proceedings of the National Academy of Sciences* 102(26):9371–9376.

Moriceau, S., and R. M. Sullivan. 2006. Maternal presence serves as a switch between learning fear and attraction in infancy. *Nature Neuroscience* 9(8):1004–1006.

Moriceau, S., K. Shionoya, K. Jakubs, and R. M. Sullivan. 2009. Early-life stress disrupts attachment learning: The role of amygdala corticosterone, locus ceruleus corticotropin releasing hormone, and olfactory bulb norepinephrine. *Journal of Neuroscience* 29(50):15745–15755.

Morris, J. C., S. E. Schindler, L. M. McCue, K. L. Moulder, T. L. S. Benzinger, C. Cruchaga, A. M. Fagan, E. Grant, B. A. Gordon, D. M. Holtzman, and C. Xiong. 2019. Assessment of racial disparities in biomarkers for Alzheimer disease. *JAMA Neurology* 76(3):264–273.

Müller, V. I., E. C. Cieslik, I. Serbanescu, A. R. Laird, P. T. Fox, and S. B. Eickhoff. 2017. Altered brain activity in unipolar depression revisited: Meta-analyses of neuroimaging studies. *JAMA Psychiatry* 74(1):47–55.

Murphy, M., K. Glaser, and E. Grundy. 1997. Marital status and long-term illness in Great Britain. *Journal of Marriage and the Family* 156–164.

Musiek, E. S. 2017. Circadian rhythms in ad pathogenesis: A critical appraisal. *Current Sleep Medicine Reports* 3(2):85–92.

Nasca, C., B. Bigio, D. Zelli, P. de Angelis, T. Lau, M. Okamoto, H. Soya, J. Ni, L. Brichta, P. Greengard, R. L. Neve, F. S. Lee, and B. S. McEwen. 2017. Role of the astroglial glutamate exchanger xct in ventral hippocampus in resilience to stress. *Neuron* 96(2):402–413.

Nasca, C., B. Bigio, F. S. Lee, S. P. Young, M. M. Kautz, A. Albright, J. Beasley, D. S. Millington, A. A. Mathé, J. H. Kocsis, J. W. Murrough, B. S. McEwen, and N. Rasgon. 2018. Acetyl-L-carnitine deficiency in patients with major depressive disorder. *Proceedings of the National Academy of Sciences* 115(34):8627–8632.

NASEM (National Academies of Sciences, Engineering, and Medicine). 2019. *The promise of adolescence: Realizing opportunity for all youth.* Washington, DC: The National Academies Press.

Nin, M. S., L. A. Martinez, F. Pibiri, M. Nelson, and G. Pinna. 2011. Neurosteroids reduce social isolation-induced behavioral deficits: A proposed link with neurosteroid-mediated upregulation of bdnf expression. *Frontiers in Endocrinology* 2:73.

NRC and IOM (National Research Council and Institute of Medicine). 2000. *From neurons to neighborhoods: The science of early childhood development.* Washington, DC: National Academy Press.

Oh, H., C. Madison, S. Baker, G. Rabinovici, and W. Jagust. 2016. Dynamic relationships between age, amyloid-β deposition, and glucose metabolism link to the regional vulnerability to Alzheimer's disease. *Brain: A Journal of Neurology* 139(Pt 8):2275–2289.

Oman, D., C. E. Thoresen, and K. McMahon. 1999. Volunteerism and mortality among the community-dwelling elderly. *Journal of Health and Psychology* 4(3):301–316.

O'Sullivan, M., D. K. Jones, P. E. Summers, R. G. Morris, S. C. Williams, and H. S. Markus. 2001. Evidence for cortical "disconnection" as a mechanism of age-related cognitive decline. *Neurology* 57(4):632–638.

Ott, S. R., and S. M. Rogers. 2010. Gregarious desert locusts have substantially larger brains with altered proportions compared with the solitarious phase. *Proceedings. Biological Sciences* 277(1697):3087–3096.

Palva, J. M., S. Monto, S. Kulashekhar, and S. Palva. 2010. Neuronal synchrony reveals working memory networks and predicts individual memory capacity. *Proceedings of the National Academy of Sciences* 107(16):7580–7585.

Park, D. C., and P. Reuter-Lorenz. 2009. The adaptive brain: Aging and neurocognitive scaffolding. *Annual Review of Psychology* 60:173–196.

Peplau, L., D. Russell, and M. Heim. 1979. The experience of loneliness. In *New approaches to social problems: Applications of attribution theory*. Edited by I. H. Frieze, D. Bar-Tal, and J. S. Carroll. San Francisco, CA: Jossey-Bass.

Perissinotto, C. M., I. Stijacic Cenzer, and K. E. Covinsky. 2012. Loneliness in older persons: A predictor of functional decline and death. *Archives of Internal Medicine* 172(14):1078–1083.

Poldrack, R. A., T. O. Laumann, O. Koyejo, B. Gregory, A. Hover, M.-Y. Chen, K. J. Gorgolewski, J. Luci, S. J. Joo, R. L. Boyd, S. Hunicke-Smith, Z. B. Simpson, T. Caven, V. Sochat, J. M. Shine, E. Gordon, A. Z. Snyder, B. Adeyemo, S. E. Petersen, D. C. Glahn, D. Reese Mckay, J. E. Curran, H. H. H. Göring, M. A. Carless, J. Blangero, R. Dougherty, A. Leemans, D. A. Handwerker, L. Frick, E. M. Marcotte, and J. A. Mumford. 2015. Long-term neural and physiological phenotyping of a single human. *Nature Communications* 6(1):8885.

Poldrack, R. A., G. Huckins, and G. Varoquaux. 2019. Establishment of best practices for evidence for prediction: A review. *JAMA Psychiatry*. [Epub ahead of print].

Power, J. D., A. L. Cohen, S. M. Nelson, G. S. Wig, K. A. Barnes, J. A. Church, A. C. Vogel, T. O. Laumann, F. M. Miezin, B. L. Schlaggar, and S. E. Petersen. 2011. Functional network organization of the human brain. *Neuron* 72(4):665–678.

Power, J. D., A. Mitra, T. O. Laumann, A. Z. Snyder, B. L. Schlaggar, and S. E. Petersen. 2014. Methods to detect, characterize, and remove motion artifact in resting state fMRI. *NeuroImage* 84:320–341.

Pressman, S. D., S. Cohen, G. E. Miller, A. Barkin, B. S. Rabin, and J. J. Treanor. 2005. Loneliness, social network size, and immune response to influenza vaccination in college freshmen. *Health Psychology* 24(3):297–306.

Ram, G. 2015. Growth curve modeling and longitudinal factor analysis. In *Handbook of child psychology and developmental science*. Hoboken, NJ: Wiley. Pp. 1–31.

Rao, H., L. Betancourt, J. M. Giannetta, N. L. Brodsky, M. Korczykowski, B. B. Avants, J. C. Gee, J. Wang, H. Hurt, J. A. Detre, and M. J. Farah. 2010. Early parental care is important for hippocampal maturation: Evidence from brain morphology in humans. *NeuroImage* 49(1):1144–1150.

Rasgon, N., and L. Jarvik. 2004. Insulin resistance, affective disorders, and Alzheimer's disease: Review and hypothesis. *Journals of Gerontology: Series A* 59(2):M178–M183.

Rasgon, N. L., and B. S. McEwen. 2016. Insulin resistance—a missing link no more. *Molecular Psychiatry* 21(12):1648–1652.

Rasgon, N., L. Altshuler, L. Fairbanks, J. Dunkin, C. Davtyan, S. Elman, and A. Rapkin. 2002. Estrogen replacement therapy in the treatment of major depressive disorder in perimenopausal women. *Journal of Clinical Psychiatry* 63(Suppl 7):45–48.

Rasgon, N. L., H. A. Kenna, T. E. Wroolie, R. Kelley, D. Silverman, J. Brooks, K. E. Williams, B. N. Powers, J. Hallmayer, and A. Reiss. 2011. Insulin resistance and hippocampal volume in women at risk for Alzheimer's disease. *Neurobiology of Aging* 32(11):1942–1948.

Rasgon, N. L., H. A. Kenna, T. E. Wroolie, K. E. Williams, B. N. DeMuth, and D. H. Silverman. 2014. Insulin resistance and medial prefrontal gyrus metabolism in women receiving hormone therapy. *Psychiatry Research* 223(1):28–36.

Raz, N., F. M. Gunning, D. Head, J. H. Dupuis, J. McQuain, S. D. Briggs, W. J. Loken, A. E. Thornton, and J. D. Acker. 1997. Selective aging of the human cerebral cortex observed in vivo: Differential vulnerability of the prefrontal gray matter. *Cerebral Cortex* 7(3):268–282.

Rilling, J., D. Gutman, T. Zeh, G. Pagnoni, G. Berns, and C. Kilts. 2002. A neural basis for social cooperation. *Neuron* 35(2):395–405.

Rivera, H. M., K. J. Christiansen, and E. L. Sullivan. 2015. The role of maternal obesity in the risk of neuropsychiatric disorders. *Frontiers in Neuroscience* 9:194.

Roenneberg, T., T. Kuehnle, P. P. Pramstaller, J. Ricken, M. Havel, A. Guth, and M. Merrow. 2004. A marker for the end of adolescence. *Current Biology* 14(24):R1038–R1039.

Rogers, S. M., and S. R. Ott. 2015. Differential activation of serotonergic neurons during short- and long-term gregarization of desert locusts. *Proceedings of the Royal Society B: Biological Sciences* 282(1800):20142062.

Rosenberg, M., S. Noonan, J. DeGutis, and M. Esterman. 2013. Sustaining visual attention in the face of distraction: A novel gradual-onset continuous performance task. *Attention, Perception, and Psychophysics* 75(3):426–439.

Rosenberg, M. D., E. S. Finn, D. Scheinost, X. Papademetris, X. Shen, R. T. Constable, and M. M. Chun. 2016a. A neuromarker of sustained attention from whole-brain functional connectivity. *Nature Neuroscience* 19:165.

Rosenberg, M. D., S. Zhang, W.-T. Hsu, D. Scheinost, E. S. Finn, X. Shen, R. T. Constable, C.-S. R. Li, and M. M. Chun. 2016b. Methylphenidate modulates functional network connectivity to enhance attention. *Journal of Neuroscience* 36(37):9547.

Rosenberg, M. D., E. S. Finn, D. Scheinost, R. T. Constable, and M. M. Chun. 2017. Characterizing attention with predictive network models. *Trends in Cognitive Sciences* 21(4):290–302.

Rosenberg, M. D., B. J. Casey, and A. J. Holmes. 2018. Prediction complements explanation in understanding the developing brain. *Nature Communications* 9(1):589.

Rosenberg, M. D., S. A. Martinez, K. M. Rapuano, M. I. Conley, A. O. Cohen, M. D. Cornejo, D. J. Hagler, Jr., K. M. Anderson, T. D. Wager, E. Feczko, E. Earl, D. A. Fair, D. M. Barch, R. Watts, and B. J. Casey. 2019. Behavioral and neural signatures of working memory in childhood. *bioRxiv*, published online June 6.

Rosenberg, M. D., D. Scheinost, A. S. Greene, E. W. Avery, Y. H. Kwon, E. S. Finn, R. Ramani, M. Qiu, R. T. Constable, and M. M. Chun. 2020. Functional connectivity predicts changes in attention observed across minutes, days, and months. *Proceedings of the National Academy of Sciences* 117(7):3797–3807.

Russo, S. J., J. W. Murrough, M.-H. Han, D. S. Charney, and E. J. Nestler. 2012. Neurobiology of resilience. *Nature Neuroscience* 15(11):1475–1484.

Salehi, M., A. S. Greene, A. Karbasi, X. Shen, D. Scheinost, and R. T. Constable. 2020. There is no single functional atlas even for a single individual: Functional parcel definitions change with task. *NeuroImage* 208:116366.

Sali, A. W., S. M. Courtney, and S. Yantis. 2016. Spontaneous fluctuations in the flexible control of covert attention. *Journal of Neuroscience* 36(2):445–454.

Sapolsky, R. M., S. C. Alberts, and J. Altmann. 1997. Hypercortisolism associated with social subordinance or social isolation among wild baboons. *Archives in General Psychiatry* 54(12):1137–1143.

Satterthwaite, T. D., D. H. Wolf, G. Erus, K. Ruparel, M. A. Elliott, E. D. Gennatas, R. Hopson, C. Jackson, K. Prabhakaran, W. B. Bilker, M. E. Calkins, J. Loughead, A. Smith, D. R. Roalf, H. Hakonarson, R. Verma, C. Davatzikos, R. C. Gur, and R. E. Gur. 2013. Functional maturation of the executive system during adolescence. *Journal of Neuroscience* 33(41):16249–16261.

Satterthwaite, T. D., M. A. Elliott, K. Ruparel, J. Loughead, K. Prabhakaran, M. E. Calkins, R. Hopson, C. Jackson, J. Keefe, M. Riley, F. D. Mentch, P. Sleiman, R. Verma, C. Davatzikos, H. Hakonarson, R. C. Gur, and R. E. Gur. 2014. Neuroimaging of the Philadelphia neurodevelopmental cohort. *NeuroImage* 86:544–553.

Savalia, N. K., P. F. Agres, M. Y. Chan, E. J. Feczko, K. M. Kennedy, and G. S. Wig. 2017. Motion-related artifacts in structural brain images revealed with independent estimates of in-scanner head motion. *Human Brain Mapping* 38(1):472–492.

Seaman, K. L., M. A. Gorlick, K. M. Vekaria, M. Hsu, D. H. Zald, and G. R. Samanez-Larkin. 2016. Adult age differences in decision making across domains: Increased discounting of social and health-related rewards. *Psychology and Aging* 31(7):737–746.

Seaman, K. L., N. Brooks, T. M. Karrer, J. J. Castrellon, S. F. Perkins, L. C. Dang, M. Hsu, D. H. Zald, and G. R. Samanez-Larkin. 2018. Subjective value representations during effort, probability and time discounting across adulthood. *Social Cognitive and Affective Neuroscience* 13(5):449–459.

Seaman, K. L., C. T. Smith, E. J. Juarez, L. C. Dang, J. J. Castrellon, L. L. Burgess, M. D. San Juan, P. M. Kundzicz, R. L. Cowan, D. H. Zald, and G. R. Samanez-Larkin. 2019. Differential regional decline in dopamine receptor availability across adulthood: Linear and nonlinear effects of age. *Human Brain Mapping* 40(10):3125–3138.

Shaw, E. E., A. P. Schultz, R. A. Sperling, and T. Hedden. 2015. Functional connectivity in multiple cortical networks is associated with performance across cognitive domains in older adults. *Brain Connectivity* 5(8):505–516.

Shen, X., E. S. Finn, D. Scheinost, M. D. Rosenberg, M. M. Chun, X. Papademetris, and R. T. Constable. 2017. Using connectome-based predictive modeling to predict individual behavior from brain connectivity. *Nature Protocols* 12(3):506–518.

Shine, J. M., O. Koyejo, and R. A. Poldrack. 2016. Temporal metastates are associated with differential patterns of time-resolved connectivity, network topology, and attention. *Proceedings of the National Academy of Sciences* 113(35):9888–9891.

Silk, J. B., J. C. Beehner, T. J. Bergman, C. Crockford, A. L. Engh, L. R. Moscovice, R. M. Wittig, R. M. Seyfarth, and D. L. Cheney. 2010. Strong and consistent social bonds enhance the longevity of female baboons. *Current Biology* 20(15):1359–1361.

Silvers, J. A., D. S. Lumian, L. Gabard-Durnam, D. G. Gee, B. Goff, D. S. Fareri, C. Caldera, J. Flannery, E. H. Telzer, K. L. Humphreys, and N. Tottenham. 2016. Previous institutionalization is followed by broader amygdala–hippocampal–PFC network connectivity during aversive learning in human development. *Journal of Neuroscience* 36(24):6420–6430.

Simmons, J. P., L. D. Nelson, and U. Simonsohn. 2011. False-positive psychology: Undisclosed flexibility in data collection and analysis allows presenting anything as significant. *Psychological Science* 22(11):1359–1366.

Sit, D. K., J. McGowan, C. Wiltrout, R. S. Diler, J. J. Dills, J. Luther, A. Yang, J. D. Ciolino, H. Seltman, S. R. Wisniewski, M. Terman, and K. L. Wisner. 2018. Adjunctive bright light therapy for bipolar depression: A randomized double-blind placebo-controlled trial. *American Journal of Psychiatry* 175(2):131–139.

Smilek, D., J. S. Carriere, and J. A. Cheyne. 2010. Out of mind, out of sight: Eye blinking as indicator and embodiment of mind wandering. *Psychological Science* 21(6):786–789.

Smith, T. W., J. M. Ruiz, and B. N. Uchino. 2004. Mental activation of supportive ties, hostility, and cardiovascular reactivity to laboratory stress in young men and women. *Health Psychology Journal* 23(5):476–485.

Song, J., R. M. Birn, M. Boly, T. B. Meier, V. A. Nair, M. E. Meyerand, and V. Prabhakaran. 2014. Age-related reorganizational changes in modularity and functional connectivity of human brain networks. *Brain Connectivity* 4(9):662–676.

Sowell, E. R., P. M. Thompson, C. M. Leonard, S. E. Welcome, E. Kan, and A. W. Toga. 2004. Longitudinal mapping of cortical thickness and brain growth in normal children. *Journal of Neuroscience* 24(38):8223–8231.

Spencer, R. C., D. M. Devilbiss, and C. W. Berridge. 2015. The cognition-enhancing effects of psychostimulants involve direct action in the prefrontal cortex. *Biological Psychiatry* 77(11):940–950.

Spreng, R. N., W. D. Stevens, J. D. Viviano, and D. L. Schacter. 2016. Attenuated anticorrelation between the default and dorsal attention networks with aging: Evidence from task and rest. *Neurobiology and Aging* 45:149–160.

Stein, M. B., C. Koverola, C. Hanna, M. G. Torchia, and B. McClarty. 1997. Hippocampal volume in women victimized by childhood sexual abuse. *Psychological Medicine* 27(4):951–959.

Stern, Y., B. Gurland, T. K. Tatemichi, M. X. Tang, D. Wilder, and R. Mayeux. 1994. Influence of education and occupation on the incidence of Alzheimer's disease. *JAMA* 271(13):1004–1010.

Sullivan, E. L., B. Grayson, D. Takahashi, N. Robertson, A. Maier, C. L. Bethea, M. S. Smith, K. Coleman, and K. L. Grove. 2010. Chronic consumption of a high-fat diet during pregnancy causes perturbations in the serotonergic system and increased anxiety-like behavior in nonhuman primate offspring. *Journal of Neuroscience* 30(10):3826.

Sullivan, E. L., K. F. Holton, E. K. Nousen, A. N. Barling, C. A. Sullivan, C. B. Propper, and J. T. Nigg. 2015. Early identification of ADHD risk via infant temperament and emotion regulation: A pilot study. *Journal of Child Psychology and Psychiatry* 56(9):949–957.

Szyf, M., I. C. Weaver, F. A. Champagne, J. Diorio, and M. J. Meaney. 2005. Maternal programming of steroid receptor expression and phenotype through DNA methylation in the rat. *Frontiers in Neuroendocrinology* 26(3–4):139–162.

Tang, M. X., P. Cross, H. Andrews, D. M. Jacobs, S. Small, K. Bell, C. Merchant, R. Lantigua, R. Costa, Y. Stern, and R. Mayeux. 2001. Incidence of AD in African-Americans, Caribbean Hispanics, and Caucasians in northern Manhattan. *Neurology* 56(1):49–56.

Thompson, J. R., J. C. Valleau, A. N. Barling, J. G. Franco, M. DeCapo, J. L. Bagley, and E. L. Sullivan. 2017. Exposure to a high-fat diet during early development programs behavior and impairs the central serotonergic system in juvenile non-human primates. *Frontiers in Endocrinology* 8:164.

Tottenham, N. 2012. Human amygdala development in the absence of species-expected caregiving. *Developmental Psychobiology* 54(6):598–611.

Tottenham, N., and A. Galván. 2016. Stress and the adolescent brain: Amygdala-prefrontal cortex circuitry and ventral striatum as developmental targets. *Neuroscience and Biobehavioral Reviews* 70:217–227.

Tottenham, N., T. A. Hare, A. Millner, T. Gilhooly, J. D. Zevin, and B. J. Casey. 2011. Elevated amygdala response to faces following early deprivation. *Developmental Science* 14(2):190–204.

Tottenham, N., M. Shapiro, J. Flannery, C. Caldera, and R. M. Sullivan. 2019. Parental presence switches avoidance to attraction learning in children. *Nature Human Behaviour* 3(10):1070–1077.

Toussaint, L. L., A. D. Owen, and A. Cheadle. 2012. Forgive to live: Forgiveness, health, and longevity. *Journal of Behavioral Medicine* 35(4):375–386.

Turek, F. W., C. Joshu, A. Kohsaka, E. Lin, G. Ivanova, E. McDearmon, A. Laposky, S. Losee-Olson, A. Easton, and D. R. Jensen. 2005. Obesity and metabolic syndrome in circadian clock mutant mice. *Science* 308(5724):1043–1045.

Varoquaux, G. 2018. Cross-validation failure: Small sample sizes lead to large error bars. *NeuroImage* 180(Pt A):68–77.

Volkow, N. D., L. Chang, G. J. Wang, J. S. Fowler, D. Franceschi, M. Sedler, S. J. Gatley, E. Miller, R. Hitzemann, Y. S. Ding, and J. Logan. 2001. Loss of dopamine transporters in methamphetamine abusers recovers with protracted abstinence. *Journal of Neuroscience* 21(23):9414–9418.

Vyas, A., R. Mitra, B. S. Shankaranarayana Rao, and S. Chattarji. 2002. Chronic stress induces contrasting patterns of dendritic remodeling in hippocampal and amygdaloid neurons. *Journal of Neuroscience* 22(15):6810–6818.

Waite, L. J., and E. L. Lehrer. 2003. The benefits from marriage and religion in the United States: A comparative analysis. *Population and Development Review* 29(2):255–276.

Watson, K., C. Nasca, L. Aasly, B. McEwen, and N. Rasgon. 2018. Insulin resistance, an unmasked culprit in depressive disorders: Promises for interventions. *Neuropharmacology* 136(Pt B):327–334.

Wehr, T. A. 2018. Bipolar mood cycles associated with lunar entrainment of a circadian rhythm. *Translational Psychiatry* 8(1):151.

Werker, J. F., and T. K. Hensch. 2015. Critical periods in speech perception: New directions. *Annual Review of Psychology* 66:173–196.

Wig, G. S. 2017. Segregated systems of human brain networks. *Trends in Cognitive Sciences* 21(12):981–996.

Wig, G. S., B. L. Schlaggar, and S. E. Petersen. 2011. Concepts and principles in the analysis of brain networks. *Annals of the New York Academy of Sciences* 1224:126–146.

Wilson, R. S., L. A. Beckett, L. L. Barnes, J. A. Schneider, J. Bach, D. A. Evans, and D. A. Bennett. 2002. Individual differences in rates of change in cognitive abilities of older persons. *Psychology and Aging* 17(2):179–193.

Xia, C. H., Z. Ma, R. Ciric, S. Gu, R. F. Betzel, A. N. Kaczkurkin, M. E. Calkins, P. A. Cook, A. García de la Garza, S. N. Vandekar, Z. Cui, T. M. Moore, D. R. Roalf, K. Ruparel, D. H. Wolf, C. Davatzikos, R. C. Gur, R. E. Gur, R. T. Shinohara, D. S. Bassett, and T. D. Satterthwaite. 2018. Linked dimensions of psychopathology and connectivity in functional brain networks. *Nature Communications* 9(1):3003.

Zahodne, L. B., J. J. Manly, A. Narkhede, E. Y. Griffith, C. DeCarli, N. S. Schupf, R. Mayeux, and A. M. Brickman. 2015. Structural MRI predictors of late-life cognition differ across African Americans, Hispanics, and whites. *Current Alzheimer Research* 12(7):632–639.

Zahodne, L. B., J. J. Manly, M. Azar, A. M. Brickman, and M. M. Glymour. 2016. Racial disparities in cognitive performance in mid- and late adulthood: Analyses of two cohort studies. *Journal of the American Geriatrics Society* 64(5):959–964.

Zonneveld, H. I., R. H. Pruim, D. Bos, H. A. Vrooman, R. L. Muetzel, A. Hofman, S. A. Rombouts, A. van der Lugt, W. J. Niessen, M. A. Ikram, and M. W. Vernooij. 2019. Patterns of functional connectivity in an aging population: The Rotterdam study. *NeuroImage* 189:432–444.